The Knowing of Woman's Kind in Childing

MEDIEVAL WOMEN: TEXTS AND CONTEXTS

4

The Knowing of Woman's Kind in Childing

A Middle English Version of Material Derived from the Trotula and Other Sources

edited by

Alexandra Barratt

MEDIEVAL WOMEN: TEXTS AND CONTEXTS

4

BREPOLS

British Library Cataloguing in Publication Data

The knowing of woman's kind in childing: a Middle English version of
    material derived from the Trotula and other sources. - (Medieval women :
    texts and contexts ; 4)
    1.Childbirth - Early works to 1800 2. Medicine, Medieval - Sources
    I.Barratt, Alexandra
    618.2'0902

ISBN 2503510736

© 2001 Brepols Publishers n.v., Turnhout, Belgium

D/2001/0095/85
ISBN 2-503-51073-6

Printed in the EU on acid-free paper.

Contents

Preface

My primary debt, as will be obvious from the footnotes, is to Monica Green and her work on the Latin and vernacular Trotula texts. Without her own scholarly work, her personal assistance, and her enthusiasm this edition would never have come into existence. I should also like to thank Margaret Burrell, Barbara Newman, Païvi Pahta, Linda Voigts and Jocelyn Wogan-Browne for help, encouragement, and advice.

Some of the work for this edition was carried out while I was Visiting Professor at the Centre for Medieval Studies, University of York. I wish to thank Professor Mark Ormrod, the Director, and Professor Felicity Riddy for their hospitality and their interest in my work, and also my own university, the University of Waikato, whose generous study leave policies made it possible at all. In addition, the former University of Waikato School of Humanities Research Committee made available a grant to enable me to examine manuscripts in the British Library in 1999, for which I must thank them.

I also acknowledge the assistance of staff in the various libraries where I have worked, in particular the Bodleian Library, the Cambridge University Library, the British Library, and, of course, the University of Waikato.

Finally I wish to thank my husband, Robert A. S. Welch, for his support and his twenty-first-century perspective on his scientific predecessors, particularly for his interest in early methods of sperm-sexing and his explanation of the reproductive systems of pigs and cows and their possible relevance to the theory of the seven-chambered womb.

.

Abbreviations

BL	British Library, London
BN	Bibliothèque Nationale, Paris
CUL	Cambridge University Library
DMLBS	*Dictionary of Medieval Latin from British Sources*, prepared by R. E. Latham (London: British Academy, 1975–)
IMEV	Carleton Brown and Rossell Hope Robbins, *The Index of Middle English Verse* (New York: Medieval Academy, 1943)
LALME	*A Linguistic Atlas of Late Mediaeval English*, ed. by Angus McIntosh, M. L. Samuels, Michael Benskin, with the assistance of Margaret Laing and Keith Williamson, 4 vols. (Aberdeen: Aberdeen University Press, 1986)
Lat.	Latin
Lewis & Short	*A Latin Dictionary*, ed. by Charlton T. Lewis and Charles Short (Oxford: Clarendon Press, 1879, repr. 1962)

ME   Middle English

MED   *Middle English Dictionary,* ed. by Hans Kurath, Sherman Kuhn and Robert E. Lewis (Ann Arbor: University of Michigan Press, 1952–)

OED   Oxford English Dictionary

(O)Fr.   (Old) French

RMLWL   *Revised Medieval Latin Word-List from British and Irish Sources,* prepared by R. E. Latham under the direction of a committee appointed by the British Academy (London: Oxford University Press, 1965)

Summary Catalogue   *A Summary Catalogue of Western Manuscripts in the Bodleian Library at Oxford,* 7 vols. (Oxford: Clarendon Press, 1953)

Suppl.   Carleton Brown and John L. Cutler, *Supplement to the Index of Middle English Verse* (Lexington: Kentucky University Press, 1965)

TK   Lynn Thorndike and Pearl Kibre, *A Catalogue of Incipits of Mediaeval Scientific Writings in Latin* (Cambridge, MA: Mediaeval Academy of America, rev. edn 1963)

CHAPTER ONE

General Introduction

The Text and Its Readers

The Knowing of Woman's Kind in Childing is a late-medieval gynaecological treatise written in Middle English prose which claims to be translated from French and Latin texts (or just from Latin, according to three of the manuscripts) that in their turn derive ultimately from the Greek. It survives in five manuscripts: Oxford MS Douce 37; Oxford MS Bodley 483; Cambridge University Library MS Ii. 6. 33; British Library MS Sloane 421A; and British Library MS Additional 12195. These manuscripts are described in detail below. Apart from its contribution to our knowledge of medieval gynaecology, *The Knowing of Woman's Kind* has considerable significance as a medical text written on the subject of women for a female audience. Many Middle English texts and translations were made explicitly for a female audience, but these were usually mystical and devotional texts composed for women religious or devout laywomen. Texts written specifically for secular women are extremely rare.[1]

Its subject is, indisputably, women. The text considers women's physical

---

[1] See *The Idea of the Vernacular: An Anthology of Middle English Literary Theory 1280–1520*, ed. by J. Wogan-Browne, Nicholas Watson, and others, Exeter Medieval Texts and Studies (Exeter: University of Exeter Press, 1999), pp. 386–88, where *The Knowing of Woman's Kind* is the only text listed as explicitly written for secular women.

constitution, what makes them different from men (primarily the possession of a womb) and, in particular, the three categories of problems that the womb causes. These are childbirth and its complications; three complaints that affect the womb—uterine suffocation, precipitation (or prolapse), and prefocation (or displacement); and three types of menstrual disorder—retention, failure, or excess. From that point of view it usefully illustrates some common medieval ideas about women, such as their cold, moist nature (apparently an in-built design flaw and the ultimate source of all their troubles) and their physical vulnerability. Some other more modern stereotypes, however, it does *not* illustrate, as we shall see.

That it was written for a female audience is implicit throughout the text and explicit in the Prologue. Here the writer explains that he has translated this text out of French and Latin into English because English is the language that literate women are more likely to read. They can then pass on the information it contains to illiterate women, who therefore need not reveal their problems to men (D18–22, C18–23). (The assertion that medieval Englishwomen could not read Latin but might read English is reiterated so frequently in Middle English texts, both religious and secular, that it begins to sound as much a rhetorical commonplace or *topos* as a sober statement of socio-linguistic fact.)

Moreover, while it is true that the text discusses women in the third person (as it does men), it is implied throughout that the text itself, not just the Prologue, is designed to be read by women, even perhaps by pregnant women and new mothers themselves. For instance, at one point the translator cautions his audience about the dangers of not completely emptying the womb after childbirth:

> war euery woman that trauaylith, that whan she hath trauayled, that þat humour that is wreten heer-aftir come forth clene. (C866–67)

This is more direct than the corresponding Latin, where this advice is directed, not to the woman in labour, but to the midwife. Another example of exhortations aimed, however indirectly, at the parturient woman is as follows:

> And yf hit so be-fall þat hit [the secundine] be goon to þe bottvm of þe matrys, sche þat ys delyuyrd, lett here forsse all that sche can for to put hyt forth. (D442–44)

Similarly, if the new mother has post-partum problems, she is told:

> yf hit so be here matrys go to hy when sche hath chyldydde, let hare parch otys in a panne & mak hem hote & as hote as sche may suffyre, put hem in a

bagge & bynde hem to here wombe. (D569–72)

There are other occasions, too, when the text seems to be addressing the mother. For who except the mother (or possibly the father) would be responsible for choosing a wet-nurse?

Yiff ye take a norys to your child, se that she be yonge and in good state .... (C477–78)

The wet-nurse is indirectly exhorted to watch her diet, but it is the reader of the treatise who, as her employer, is advised:

yf þe norse be to habvndant of mylk, let put here to gret labore of body so þat be labor sche may be a-swagyd. (D525–27)

The more usual address to the reader is as someone who is assisting the patient, while the patient adopts a passive rather than proactive role. For instance, from C377 onwards there is a long passage describing a variety of possible malpresentations that begins:

Yif so be the childe shewe first his hed and the remanent of the body cleue to the syde, than puttith to youre hand and dresse hym that both his handis ly joyntly to his sydes, so that he may come right foorth ....

In the Latin text from which this derives all these instructions are addressed to the midwife, but obliquely in the third person, whereas in the Middle English they are addressed directly to the second person. The translation, as here, consistently uses the plural or respectful personal pronouns *ye/yow*. The person or persons thus addressed must surely be female as they are directly and intimately involved in the birth process. Here, for instance, they insert their hands into the womb to manipulate the child; later they cut and tie the umbilical cord.

These birth attendants are also presumably literate. They must be able not only to read the text's instructions and recipes, but also to write out the brief charm given at D369–71 and, apparently, the complete text of the Magnificat (no doubt in Latin) as at D372–73. They are also not expected to take every-thing on trust and are even encouraged to show an intelligent interest in what, in the Middle Ages, passed for scientific method. Hence, perhaps, the passage where the author suggests how the efficacy of one of the recipes might be demonstrated:

Tak a tode .... And ȝif ye woll preve hit, tak & hange þat poudyre a-bouth a hennys nek to dayes by-forre ye sle here & þan draw of hare hede & sche schall not blede. (D636–41)

Apparently they should be women of some education, able to recognize Galen as a medical authority (his name is dropped, without gloss or explanation, at DC694), as well as Hippocrates, Cleopatra, and the mysterious Fabina Prycyll (or Fabyan Prycelle). And at the end of the treatise (DC1013 seq.) they are instructed in medical problems—apostemes—that affect men as well as women, although it is here that the implied audience seems to become male when the translator writes, 'a man schall do curys to hem by no cuttynge ne by no fyere' (D1068–69; C1066–67).

Apart from the constant address in the second person, there are also some third-person exhortations to 'þe mydwyffe': 'let þe mydwyffe helpe' (D376); 'let þe myddewyffe whete hare handys' (D388); 'yf þe secundynne be holdon with þe matryce, þan let þe mydwyffe draw hit forth a lytyll to þe on syde & a lytyll to þe oþyre' (D444–46). But it is not really possible, although it is tempting, to argue that the text is consistently addressed to a literate woman, not herself a professional midwife although having under her control a professional but illiterate midwife.

It seems clear enough, then, that the author and/or translator intended this text to be read primarily by, and secondarily to, women. It may even have been a woman who commissioned him to make the translation. But as to whether the text was in fact used by women, there is little direct evidence. It may well have been, but such a text would not necessarily be confined to a female readership. While one might think that it would be of no interest to men, there is ample evidence that in the Middle Ages men regularly read such treatises (and practised gynaecology).[2] The translator certainly foresaw that some might take a prurient interest in the contents, and he warns them off in no uncertain terms, in the name of the Virgin Mary ('in ovre Lady behalue') in his prologue (DC24–31).

In two manuscripts there is some textual evidence that the versions might have been produced, or modified, for particular women to read. BL MS Additional appears to have a parenthetical apostrophe to 'my ladye' towards the end (note to D1020). More convincing and of greater interest is BL MS Sloane's addition to the sentence, 'I haue this drawen and wreten it in Inglish', of the phrase '& at the pleasure of my ladye' (note to C22–23),

---

[2] See for instance Peter Murray Jones, 'Thomas Fayreford: An English Fifteenth-Century Medical Practitioner', in *Medicine from the Black Death to the French Disease*, ed. by Roger French and others (Aldershot: Ashgate, 1998), pp. 156–83, which gives evidence for Fayreford's treatment of at least twelve women for gynaecological conditions. (I am grateful to Monica Green for this reference.)

although it is possible that this refers to the Virgin rather than a secular mistress.

We have no external evidence about the ownership of any of the manuscripts, except for BL MS Additional, which may well have belonged to a house of Augustinian canons in North Creake, Norfolk. But from internal, physical evidence it is possible to argue that both Oxford MS Douce 37, CUL MS Ii. 6. 33 and BL MS Sloane 421A were designed to be used by midwives or women interested in midwifery. These questions of possible ownership are discussed in detail in Chapter Three.

The Sources

Attempts to gender the authorship of this text are likely to be even more inconclusive. The text is a translation, and there can be little doubt that the translator was a man, as were almost all medieval translators. It is true that there was at least one well-documented woman translator in early fifteenth-century England, but as far as we know she translated devotional treatises only, and only those originally written in French.[3]

But one of the sources for *The Knowing of Woman's Kind* was a text that in the Middle Ages was generally attributed, in its Latin version, to 'Trotula'. Medieval writers believed that 'Trotula' was the name of a midwife or gynaecologist from Salerno in southern Italy, who had written extensively on women's ailments, childbirth, and beauty care. Subsequently there has been much scholarly debate over whether such a woman ever existed. Recent work shows that she did indeed exist, although her name was Trota, Trotta, or Trocta, and that she was credited with a gynaecological treatise, the *De curis mulierum*, which became closely associated with two other texts not by her.[4] All three however became very popular and were widely disseminated.

The Knowing of Woman's Kind never mentions Trotula or Trota by name, though it does cite a recipe used by a lady of Salerno. But large sections of it ultimately derive, through an Old French translation,[5] from a version of the

---

[3] See Alexandra Barratt, 'Dame Eleanor Hull: a fifteenth-century translator', in *The Medieval Translator*, ed. by Roger Ellis (Cambridge: D. S. Brewer, 1989), pp. 87–101, and 'Hull [née Malet], Eleanor, Lady Hull', *New Dictionary of National Biography* (Oxford: Oxford University Press, forthcoming).

[4] See Monica H. Green, 'The Development of the Trotula', *Revue d'Histoire des Textes*, 26 (1996), 119–203, esp. p. 153.

[5] Called 'French 2 Redaction I' by Monica H. Green, 'A Handlist of Latin and

Liber de Sinthomatibus Mulierum (*LSM* 1), the first element in the so-called Trotula ensemble.[6] The attribution to 'Trotula' often occurs in its Latin title so it is at least fair to say that many people in the Middle Ages must have regarded it as coming from the pen of a woman. And even in its original, Latin, form the author claims to have written the text specifically for women:

> Therefore, their misfortune, which ought to be pitied, and especially the influence of a certain woman stirring my heart, have impelled me to give a clear explanation regarding their diseases in caring for their health.[7]

Our Middle English translator, however, did not use *LSM* 1 directly but rather worked from an Old French translation of the Latin. The Old French version used here for purposes of comparison (though probably not the copy used by the translator) is that found in London BL MS Sloane 3525, fols 246vb–253vb.[8] None of the three surviving manuscripts of the Old French contains a complete translation of the Latin, whose complex evolution and antecedents have been thoroughly discussed by Green, but are not relevant to us here.[9] We might note, however, that the only two extant copies of *LSM* 1 were both produced in England.[10] The English translator makes extensive use, in full or in part, of about two-thirds of this French text. These borrowings are recorded in the Commentary to this edition, from which it will be clear that he does not use this material slavishly. On the contrary, he rearranges it considerably, for reasons that remain obscure: his own structure

---

Vernacular Manuscripts of the so-called *Trotula* Texts Part II: The Vernacular Translations and Latin Re-Writings', *Scriptorium*, 51 (1997), 81–104 (pp. 90–91).

[6] An edition of the ensemble, together with a modern English translation, is now available: see *The 'Trotula': A Medieval Compendium of Women's Medicine*, ed. and trans. by Monica H. Green (Philadelphia: University of Pennsylvania Press, 2001). A transcription of *LSM* 1 from Oxford MS Bodley 361 is to be found in Tony Hunt, *Anglo-Norman Medicine: Volume II, Shorter Treatises* (Cambridge: D. S.Brewer, 1997), pp. 116–128.

[7] *The 'Trotula'*, ed. and trans. Green, 'Book on the Conditions of Women', [2].

[8] See Green, 'Handlist', pp. 90–91 for a description of BL MS Sloane 3525, also described by Paul Meyer, 'Manuscrits médicaux en Français', *Romania*, 44 (1915–17), 161–213 (pp. 182–214). There are three surviving manuscripts of French 2 Redaction I, one of them 'heavily abridged'.

[9] See Green, 'Handlist', esp. pp. 127–33.

[10] Green, 'Handlist', p. 133. They are found in Oxford MS Bodl. 361 (dated 1453–59), which is described further below, and Oxford Magdalen College MS lat. 173 (early fourteenth-century).

is not noticeably any more rational than that of his source. Moreover, he can be observed from time to time to adapt, or rather censor, his source in other ways as well. This is considered in greater detail in the Textual Introduction and also in the Commentary.[11]

The other major source for *The Knowing of Woman's Kind* is a Latin epitome of a text by the North African Muscio, known as *Non omnes quidem*. In the second century AD the Hellenistic Greek physician Soranus had written a gynaecological treatise, the *Gynaecia*, which was to prove extremely influential in Western Europe.[12] In the sixth century (probably) Muscio, of whom we otherwise know nothing, composed a Latin version of this, specifically for non-Greek speaking midwives, with the incipit 'Cum frequentius nobis in mulieribus obstetrix necessaria'.[13] (Soranus' Greek text had also been translated into Latin by Caelius Aurelianus, but our Middle English text shows no signs of any contact with that version.) Some time in or before the twelfth century (the date of the earliest surviving manuscript) an adaptation or epitome of Muscio's text was made. This is known, from its opening words, as *Non omnes quidem*. Hanson and Green list nine known manuscripts, ranging in date from the early twelfth to the fifteenth century.[14] For the purposes of this edition, we have used the version found in Oxford Bodley MS Laud Misc. 567, fols 62–66v, a manuscript which is described in detail below.

The Middle English translator seems to have worked directly from the Latin text in this case, as there is no known Old French version as such. But the rendering of the Latin is fairly free, so there may well have been a French intermediary that has not survived. (In contrast, the Middle English

---

[11] See also Alexandra Barratt, 'Translation and Censorship in a Middle English Gynaecological Treatise', in *The Medieval Translator / Traduire au Moyen Age*, ed. by Roger Ellis, René Tixier, and Bernd Weitemeier (Turnhout: Brepols, 1998), pp. 306–320.

[12] See Ann Ellis Hanson and Monica H. Green, 'Soranus of Ephesus: *Methodicorum princeps*', in *Aufstieg und Niedergang der Römischen Welt / Rise and Decline of the Roman World*, ed. by Wolfganag Haase and Hildegard Temporini, Part II, Vol. 37.2 (Berlin and New York: Walter de Gruyter), 968–1075 (pp. 1042–61), for an authoritative account of the influence of Soranus.

[13] This text was edited from the three known manuscripts in the nineteenth century: see *Sorani Gynaeciorum Vetus Translatio Latina*, ed. by Valentine Rose (Leipzig: Teubner, 1882).

[14] See Hanson and Green, 'Soranus of Ephesus', p. 1074.

translation of the French version of *LSM* 1 is very close and literal.) Out of the first fifty-eight chapters of *Non omnes quidem*, he makes use of three extensive blocks of text. But he does not necessarily use complete runs of chapters nor does he always keep the chapters in the order in which they appear in the Latin. In fact, he rearranges this material even more radically than the Trotula material, again for reasons that are unclear.

Some interesting cultural shifts take place in the use of the *Non omnes quidem* material. These pointedly illustrate the dangers of using the Middle English text as unproblematized evidence for actual gynaecological practice in England in the fifteenth century. Some of the material in the Middle English text in fact goes straight back to Soranus, to the quite different world of second-century Imperial Rome. Two simple examples: the English includes a section on which newborns will be easy to rear—those born at full term after an easy pregnancy, and who are lively and responsive. If we trace the history of this belief back through *Non omnes quidem* to Soranus, we find very similar criteria. But Soranus is concerned with those babies worth rearing at all, infanticide being a common practice in Rome. Another example: the English text advises the midwife to cut the umbilical cord with a sharp knife or a razor and not with glass, a piece of pottery or a sharp stone. The latter practice is condemned as 'þe folly of sume olde women' and as 'wyche-crafte' (DC460–63). One might think this provided valuable evidence of a common late-medieval English folk practice, but once again this passage goes back, virtually unchanged, to Soranus.

The translator also takes some recipes from a third source, the *Genicia Cleopatrae ad Theodotam*, a Latin text attributed to Cleopatra (traditionally identified with the Egyptian queen) and often found in manuscripts with *Non omnes quidem*. There is probably at least one further source that has not been traced, although some of the text may well be the medieval English translator's own original contribution. In particular the section on the differences between men and women is quite different in outlook from the prologue that it immediately follows. The prologue, derived from the Trotula text, constructs sex differences in terms of the 'primary qualities' of Galen: men are hot and dry, women are cold and moist. But this theory, widespread in the Middle Ages, does not rate a mention in the description of the 'v dyuersiteys be-tven man & woman' (DC40–41): the differences enumerated are purely empirical and no attempt is made to theorize them. Indeed, they could well be the result of personal observation, and they are accurate enough as far as they go. So quite possibly this is the translator's own contribution.

This section has another point of interest. It is highly original in its even-handedness, and consequently it does not fit our own modern stereotypes about the significance of male-female differences. It is virtually an article of faith in some quarters that the female is defined in terms of lack, but this text defines women in terms of what they possess, in particular the 'maryce' or uterus. In enumerating each of the first four differences, male and female characteristics are mentioned. But in the fifth, only women are cited as possessing a distinctive organ and it is the man who is defined in terms of lack: 'þer hath sche a vessyll þat no man hath' (D50–51; C49–50).

No source has been found for the translation's discussion of nutrition and digestion (D187–203), of respiration and of the heat-seeking tendencies of the womb (D141–52), or even of a passing comment about pores (D503–05). If these are the translator's own contributions, he (or she) may well have had a strong interest specifically in anatomy and physiology, although he shows no signs of any practical experience in this area. Indeed, he is happy to retail the fanciful theory of the seven-chambered womb (see Commentary). The story, however, about the baby who was safely delivered although his hands and feet were joined (D425–28) might well derive from personal experience as a practising obstetrician.

In conclusion it should be emphasized that this text is somewhat different from the usual run of Middle English translations. Its adaptor or compiler—such terms are perhaps more appropriate than mere 'translator'—seems to have shown a remarkable amount of discrimination, both in searching out his sources, in selecting and combining them, and in possibly adding his own material. Such an approach is very far from the careful, often slavish, word-for-word translation style favoured by many in medieval England.

CHAPTER TWO

The Manuscripts

Manuscripts of the Middle English Texts

The treatise is extant in five manuscripts, described below:

1. Oxford Bodley MS Douce 37 (SC 21611)

Described by the *Summary Catalogue* as follows: 'In English, on parchment; written in the first half of the 15th cent.: $5^{3/8}$ x $3^{7/8}$ in., iv + 42 leaves. A treatise on the diseases of women'. Also described by Laurel Braswell, *Index of Middle English Prose Handlist IV: A Handlist of Douce Manuscripts containing Middle English Prose in the Bodleian Library, Oxford* (Cambridge: D. S. Brewer, 1987), pp. 12–13, though with many errors in the transcriptions of the incipit and explicit; and by Monica H. Green, 'Obstetrical and Gynecological Texts in Middle English', *Studies in the Age of Chaucer*, 14 (1992), 53–88 (pp. 67–68), and 'A Handlist of Latin and Vernacular Manuscripts of the So-called *Trotula* Texts. Part II: The Vernacular Translations and Latin Re-writings', *Scriptorium*, 51 (1997), 80-104 (p. 86).

Fols i–iii are paper, fols iv–end are parchment.

Collation: $1-4^8$, 5^7; catchwords at the end of the first two quires.

Fol. 1r is considerably rubbed and faded, as if the booklet had circulated unbound for some time. Regularly 22 lines to the pages; some underlinings in pale red ink; some marginal notes and annotations in a later hand; on fol. iv a post-medieval (?seventeenth-century) hand has written 'A Treatise of Womens Distemper'.

Contains only one text, *The Knowing of Woman's Kind in Childing* (though not given this or any other title), fols 1–37v: *inc.* '[O]Vre lorde god whan he had storid þe worlde of all creaturis he made manne & woman', *expl.* '& þan a man schall do curys to hem by no cuttynge ne by no fyere.' Followed without a break by seven gynaecological recipes (fols 37v–39r), *inc.* 'Tak schepys dong & poudyre of comyn', *expl.* '& gyf þer of at onys to þe pacient jd worth or morre. Thys is to putte out þe secundine or aftyre byrth.'

Green suggests that, as this text is the only one in the codex, it 'conceivably could have circulated independently among midwives or laywomen with medical interests'.[1] The manuscript's compact size also suggests that it was designed for practical use, being small enough to be conveniently carried around to the bedsides of women in labour.

2. Oxford MS Bodley 483 (SC 2062)

Described by the *Summary Catalogue* as follows: 'In English, on paper: written in two hands about the middle of the 15th cent.: 9 x 6$^{1/2}$ in., 117 leaves.' An extensive collection or compendium of herbal, medical and gynaecological treatises in prose and verse, all in English. Also described by Green, 'Obstetrical and Gynecological Texts', p. 67, and 'A Handlist', pp. 85–86. She notes the inscription 'Jhon Barcke' in a hand of *c.* 1500 on fol. 117v, and that the manuscript was 'probably owned in the later sixteenth century by John Twynne of Canterbury', citing Andrew G. Watson, 'John Twynne of Canterbury (d. 1581) as a Collector of Medieval Manuscripts: A Preliminary Investigation', *The Library*, 6th ser., 8 (1986), p. 151.

Collation: 1^{10} (lacks 1, 10); 2^{10}; 3^{6}; 4-9^{8}; 10-11^{10}; 12^{10} (lacks 7, 8, 9). In spite of the three missing leaves in the final quire, there is no lacuna in the text, suggesting that they might have been written in error or spoiled in some way and removed before the manuscript was bound.

Texts written by Hand 1 vary between 28 and 29 lines per page, texts by Hand 2 from 23 to 25 lines per page.

---

[1] 'Obstetrical and Gynecological Texts', p. 59.

Contents:

1. Series of general medical recipes, fols 1–13; *inc.* (acephalous, lacks first leaf) '... aliam tria grana mirre ante accessum febriis'.
2. Prose herbary, arranged alphabetically, fols 14–51; *inc.* 'Agnus castus is an herbe that men clepyth Toutsayn or parke leves'. On fol. 18 there is a change of hand and of ink (from brown to black).
3. Poem on the virtues of the herb rosemary, fols 51–54; *inc.* 'As yn boke wrytyn y fynde off doctors yn dyuerse londe', *expl.* 'Bynde hit on thy navyl all a bowt/ And hit shall staunge some wit ow3t dow3t'. An extract from *IMEV* 3754 (see also Suppl.), but this manuscript is not listed there.
4. Continuation of alphabetical herbary (Item 2), fols 54–57, with *saturyon, salgia, savina.*
5. Another prose herbary, fols 57–80; *inc.* 'Here men may se the virtues off herbes wyche ben hot & colde and for how many thynggis they ben gode After plato galyen & ypocras', *expl.* '& a noynte þe yen that beth dymme & hit shall clere them'.

Fols 80v–81v blank.

6. *The Knowing of Woman's Kind in Childing,* fols 82–103v; *inc.* 'Our lord god when he had stored the worlde of all creatours he made man & woman', *expl.* 'and then a man shall doo cure hem by no cuttyng ne by no fyer'. Followed without a break (fols 103v–104v) by seven gynaeco-logical recipes (as in Douce 37), *inc.* 'Take shepys dung and powder of comyne', *expl.* (fol. 104v) 'And þerof at onys gyffe to the pacient j^d worthe or more. This is to put oute the secundyne or aftyr byrthe'; reverts to Hand 1.
7. Short prose treatise on swollen testicles, fol. 104v; *inc.* 'Now here begynneth of the swellyng of ballokis the whiche other whyle swellyn because of humours', *expl.* 'put it vpon the grevaunce'.
8. Short prose treatise on ailments of the penis, fols 105–106; *inc.* 'Now here begynneth of the grevaunce of mannys yerd', *expl.* 'after þe tente is drawen out of hyt hit is a token of helyng'.
9. Short prose treatise on involuntary ejaculation, fols 103–107; *inc.* 'De pollucione. Now here begynneth of nyght pollucion, þat is to sey that a man other whyle yeveth hys kynde in hys slepe', *expl.* 'whiche curys been tolde in þe fyrst chapitre'.
10. Short prose treatise on menstrual disorders, fol. 107; *inc.* 'De morbis mulierum. Now here begynneth þe siknesse that comyth to a woman oftest and moste kyndely longeth to hem', *expl.* 'in þe last quarter of the mone'.

11. Another treatise on menstruation, fols 107-110; *inc.* 'De Fluxu menstruorum. Now here begynneth of over muche sheddyng of womannys flowrys', *expl.* 'and this shall lett that þe flowrys shall not come downe'.

12. Short treatise on the symptoms of pregnancy, fols 110–112v; *inc.* 'Of generall tokyns of concepcion oon is this if she be conceived when she was last servyd', *expl.* 'and lighthede of hote blode than in þe lyfte halfe'.

13. Short treatise on difficulties in childbirth, fols 112v–114v; *inc.* 'Sequitur de difficultate partus mulierum. Now here begynneth of þe trauelyng that / women hauen in chylde beryng', *expl.* 'and anoon she shall be deliuered if it be hir tyme'.

14. Short treatise on the deliverance of the afterbirth, fols 114v–116; *inc.* 'Sequitur de secundina. Now here begynneth of þe childis hame whiche is clepyd secundina. Constantynus seith', *expl.* 'and these medicines been sufficient to help eny woman by the grace of god. Explicit istud Regimen. Deo gracias.'

15. Recipes in two further hands, fols 116v–117; *inc.* 'for to stoppe þe flowrys yff a woman', *expl.* 'for thys ys well provyd'.

Green comments on the codex as a whole that 'while the receptary and herbals ... may have been accessible to a lay reader, a medical specialist seems the more likely user'.[2]

3. Cambridge University Library MS Ii. 6. 33

This volume consists of two originally independent manuscripts that were bound together at an early date. Described by the Cambridge University Library catalogue as: 'A 12mo, on paper, of 71 leaves, in writing of the XVth and XVIth century'.[3] Now measures 150 x 113 mm. (6 x 4$^{1/4}$ inches). 22 or 23 lines to the page; also described by Green, 'Obstetrical and Gynecological Treatises', p. 66, and 'Hand-list', p. 85.

Section A, fols 1–32, paper, slightly different in colour from Section B and slightly larger in size, trimmed. Collation: 1^{16}, 2^{14} (lacks 3). Contains only one item, *The Book of Rota, inc.* 'This boke mad a woman named Rota of þe priue siknesses þat long to a woman with medicynal to helpe them at ther

[2] 'Obstetrical and Gynecological Texts', p. 61.

[3] *A Catalogue of the Manuscripts preserved in the Library of the University of Cambridge*, 5 vols, (Cambridge: Cambridge University Press, 1856-67), III, p. 532.

neade', *expl.* 'than take a clene bason with hote water and therin holde thi handes a wyle and thow shalt see þe wormes crepe out'. Crudely written in a large sixteenth-century hand.

Section B, fols 33–68 (also numbered originally as 1-36, the numbering used in this edition). First leaf discoloured as if the booklet had circulated unbound for some time before being bound up with Section A. According to the catalogue, 'This is well written, with red initials, &c., and 21 lines to a page ... on the last two leaves are some receipts in the same hand as #2', this latter providing evidence that the two manuscripts were combined at the time of writing *The Book of Rota* or shortly after.

Collation: $1-2^{16}$, 3^{16} (lacks 16). Decoration: large red O with pen ornamentation on fol. 1, blue H with pen ornamentation on fol. 17; red paraff marks; some words written in display script; red line-fillers; some letters touched in red; some words crossed through in red; catchwords on fols 16v and 32v and final *Explicit* written on scrolls or banderolles.

Originally contained only one item, *The Knowing of Women's Kind, inc.* 'Owre lord God when he had storid the word (*sic*) of all creatures he made man and woman', *expl.* (fol. 36v) 'and than a man shal do cure hem be no cuttynge ne be no fire'. Followed without a break by a single gynecological recipe, *inc.* 'A medycine prouyd for the white floures of wyf or maydyn', *expl.* 'and the reynes of hire bak and a litill on hir navill and wel on hir body a litill a boue hire share. Explicit.' Green suggests that as this copy of the text was 'apparently ... originally independent', like MS Douce 37, it too could have circulated among women with midwifery interests.[4] Again, the small dimensions of the manuscript, especially before it was bound together with *The Book of Rota*, suggest a practical function.

4. British Library MS Sloane 421A

Paper; 30 folios. 210 x 150 mm. ($8^{1/4}$ inches x 6 inches). The earlier system of folio numbering suggests that four leaves are missing after the end of the first text, but as each leaf is now individually mounted no conclusion can be drawn from the quiring. Written throughout in one early-sixteenth-century hand. The paper is of poor quality: it is discoloured and the writing frequently shows through from the back of the sheet. The manuscript looks

---

[4] 'Obstetrical and Gynecological Texts', p. 59.

cheap and is possibly home-made; the hand though non-calligraphic is assured enough. It contains no decoration whatsoever.

Described in the Sloane Catalogue, p. 78, and also by Green, 'Obstetrical and Gynecological Texts', p. 67, and 'Hand-list', p. 85. Early sixteenth-century (before 1530). Green comments that the only other substantial item in this manuscript is a brief 'regiment of helthe' which, 'although not directed solely to a female audience, ... is nevertheless the sort of tract on moral edification we might expect women to read'.[5]

Contains:

1. *The Knowing of Woman's Kind*, followed by the same gynaecological recipe as in CUL MS Ii. 6. 33, fols 2–25v; *inc.* 'Our lord god when he had stored the world', *expl.* 'a lytell above here share.'
2. *The Regiment of Health*, a general treatise on healthy living. fols 26–29v; *inc.* 'Nevertheles that the most hie ineffable and most glorius'; *expl.* '& drynke them with honye & water'.
3. Medical recipe, fol. 30; 'To delyuer a woman of ded child. Take blades of lekes'.

In spite of its dimensions this is a slim volume; it appears to be functional, possibly produced by a reader for his or her own use. On fol. 1 appear some notes, apparently about landholdings: the following are decipherable:

> By ye nume ....
> A littell feld 5 aker es
> Eight feld 10 a kers
> .... feld   9 a kers
> medow .... 9 a kers
> oke feld   14 a kers

5. British Library MS Additional 12195

This manuscript has been very fully described by David Thomson, *A Descriptive Catalogue of Middle English Grammatical Texts* (New York and London: Garland, 1984), pp. 193–211. See also *Catalogue of Additions to the Manuscripts in the British Museum 1841-5*, pp. 50–51; D. W. Singer, *Catalogue of Latin and Vernacular Alchemical Manuscripts in Great Britain and Ireland dating from before the XVIth century*. 3 vols in 2 (Brussels: 1928–31), III, 1030; Peter Brown and Elton D. Higgs, *Index of Middle*

---

[5] 'Obstetrical and Gynecological Texts', p. 59.

English Prose Handlist V, Additional Collection (10001–14000), British Library, London (Cambridge: D. S. Brewer, 1988), pp. 45-51; Green, 'Obstetrical and Gynecological Treatises', pp. 66–67, and 'Hand-list', p. 85; and *LALME,* pp. 1, 100.

This manuscript, a collection of theological, grammatical, medical, and astrological treatises, consists of four distinct sections, written by eleven different hands: the analysis that follows is largely indebted to Thomson, *Middle English Grammatical Texts*, pp. 210–211. Section A (fols 3–15v) is in Latin and was probably written *c.* 1477 in Oxford. But it was not bound with the others until after the sixteenth century, so is irrelevant for our purposes. Section B (fols 16–58v), also in Latin, is a collection of liturgical texts, mainly Carmelite, probably made by a friar of the Carmelite priory of Burnham Norton, near North Creake in north Norfolk. Section C (fols 59–121v) contains various texts and notes, some on grammatical topics, mainly in Latin but including one in English. Most of it was written by a certain John Leke of North Creake and later it belonged to the Vicar of Toftrees, a nearby parish. Section D (fols 122–190v) contains various alchemical, magical, and scientific treatises, including *The Knowing of Women's Kind* on fols 157r–185v. It has 'no clues as to its provenance'[6] but on linguistic grounds we may reasonably assume a Norfolk audience, probably male and religious: *LALME* assigns this section to Norfolk, describing it as 'nearly all in E. Anglian English, by several hands'.

The contents of Section D are as follows:

1. English translation of Johannes Paulinus, *Experimenta de serpente*, fols 122r–124r; *inc.* 'I Iohn Paulen whan I was in the sete of Alisawndyr', *expl.* 'þe leper xal not incresyn but abydyn euere in on astat. Explicit Experimentum de serpente.'
2. Further experiments and recipes connected with the first text, fols 124–127; *inc.* 'Also ho so wele taken the powdyr', *expl.* 'the color of þe xal abydyn on þe lettris'.
3. Treatise on natural science and astronomy, allegedly translated from Greek, fols 127v–135r; *inc.* 'Here begynys the wyse book of phylosophe and astromye', *expl.* 'And that syht xal be more peyne onto hem þan all þe peynis of helle'.
4. Treatise on characteristics of people born under different zodiac signs, fols 137–139; *inc.* 'Now it is for to declare and dotermyn (*sic*)', *expl.* 'Many thyngis he schal do' (ends abruptly).

---

[6] Thomson, *Middle English Grammatical Texts*, p. 211.

5. Eight recipes, fols 139v–141r, *inc.* 'For to make braket', *expl.* 'and al maner of wonde to anoynte'.
6. More recipes, fols 142v–143v.
7. Large collection of recipes, fols 144–156.
8. *The Knowing of Woman's Kind in Childing*, fols 157–190; *inc.* 'Her folowyth þe knowyng of womanis kynde in chyldyng. Owor lord god ...', *expl.* 'and vs it daylye tyle þat sche be hall'.
9. *The Book of Hypocras*, a medical treatise, fols 185r–190v; *inc.* 'Thys bok of Ypocras tech for to knowe be þe planetis of seknes', *expl.* 'for all manere of postemus owt warde. Explicit.'

Green comments that 'the combination of astrological and medical texts ... in the original fascicle ... suggests use by a physician who might be concerned (whatever his involvement in other aspects of the care of women) to know about the processes of birth in order to cast horoscopes.'[7]

Manuscripts of the French and Latin Sources

1. The Old French translation of *LSM* 1: BL MS Sloane 3525

This is an early fourteenth-century French manuscript from the Paris region. The lack of rubricated initials to mark the beginnings of individual texts often makes it hard to be sure where one stops and another begins, but it appears to contains about thirteen medical, gynaecological, psychological, and pharmaceutical texts in Old French translations and two collections of medical recipes. It was discussed and described by Paul Mcyer in 'Manuscrits Médicaux en Français', *Romania*, 44 (1915–17), 161–214, pp. 182–214. Of such vernacular medical manuscripts in gencral he comments:

> ils nous montrent que, de bonne heure, les practiciens préféraient le français au latin. J'imagine que les femmes qui, dès le xiie siècle, s'occupaient volontiers de médecine et de chirurgie, devaient apprécier les traits élémentaires en langue vulgaire.'[8]

Our text is found on fols 246v–253v; *inc.* 'Quant Dex nostre Seignor out le mund estoré sor totes creature', *expl.* 'iceste mecine tolt l'avortier et la

---

[7] 'Obstetrical and Gynecological Texts', p. 59.

[8] Meyer, 'Manuscrits Médicaux', p. 161.

ventosité quant feme est venue a tens d'avoir enfant'. Although this manuscript is almost certainly not the copy used by the Middle English translator, it is the fullest surviving version of the Old French text and has therefore been used for purposes of comparison in this edition. MS Sloane 3525 was probably in England in the fifteenth century, or at least belonged to an English person, as on fols 178v and 179r there are three recipes written in an English hand according to Meyer, and on fol. 259 a few lines of Latin in an English fifteenth-century hand.[9]

2. *LSM* 1: Oxford MS Bodley 361 (S.C. 2462)

Most unusually for a volume containing Latin medical texts, this is a very large luxury manuscript. Its wide margins are lavishly, not to say gaudily, decorated, and there are numerous illuminated capitals at the beginnings of most of the texts, and elaborate borders. It was written in four parts by Hermannus Zurke of Greifswald, 'partly or wholly at Salisbury, between 1453 and 1459' according to the *Summary Catalogue*. Zurke was 'a scrivener working in England who was responsible for six manuscripts dated from 1449 to 1460 … five of the codices he signed are medical'.[10] On eight occasions throughout the manuscript he records his progress, stating the day, month, and year on which he had completed each section. He wrote this manuscript (as he did several others) for Gilbert Kymer, dean of Salisbury and chancellor of the University of Oxford. Linda Voigts comments on the somewhat recherché contents of the codex:

> These texts … seem to reflect the medical concerns of transalpine continental scholars … a third of the texts … are uncommon and possibly unique.[11]

That is certainly true of *LSM* 1, of which only one other copy is known (Oxford Magdalen College MS lat. 173).

In summary the principal contents are:

1. Stephanus Arnaldus, *Dietarium* (TK 571), p. 1
2. Bartholomaeus Salernitanus, *Practica* (TK 1080), p. 113

---

[9] Meyer, 'Manuscrits Médicaux', p. 183.

[10] Linda Voigts, 'Scientific and Medical Books', in *Book Production and Publishing in Britain, 1375-1475*, ed. by J. Griffiths and D. Pearsall (Cambridge: Cambridge University Press, 1989), pp. 385-86.

[11] 'Scientific and Medical Books', p. 386.

3. Johannes de Sancto Paulo, *Practica* (TK 153), p. 203
4. *Tractatus de effectibus farmacorum* (Partium in humano) (TK 1027— unique copy), p. 331
5. Petrus de Sancto Aegidio, *Practica* (Cure omnium egritudinum) (TK 362), p. 335
6. *Experimenta Minerue*, p. 394
7. *Practica Archimathei* (Cum opus quodlibet) (TK 329), p. 400
8. *De splene et Epate et eorum passionibus* (Due vene protense sunt) (TK 471— unique copy), p. 424
9. *Introductorium in practicam medicene.* (Cogitanti michi votum vestrum) (TK 230), p. 432
10. Peter de Musanda, *De cibis et potibus infirmorum* (TK 367—unique copy), p. 444
11. *Trotula maior* (Cum auctor universitatis) i.e. *LSM* 1 (TK 284), p. 458
12. *Trotula minor* (Ut de curis and Ut mulier suauissima) (TK 1615; cf. TK 1620, 1621), p. 470
13. Ricardus Anglicus, *Compendium, Practica sive medicamenta* (TK 194, but this MS not noted), p. 493

The *Cum auctor* has been edited from this manuscript by Tony Hunt, *Anglo-Norman Medicine Vol. II: Shorter Treatises* (Cambridge: D. S. Brewer, 1997), pp. 116–28. Because of its well-documented and indisputable mid-fifteenth century date, however, this particular manuscript was obviously not the one used by the Old French translator of the text found in the thirteenth-century Sloane manuscript.

3. *Non omnes quidem* and Cleopatra, *Gynaecia*: Oxford MS Laud Misc. 567 (S.C. 1507)

This is a twelfth-century English manuscript, still with its mid-twelfth-century binding. The texts are written in brown ink with red capitals and rubrics. It contains several general medical works in Latin by, or attributed to, the medical authority Constantinus Africanus, and a small clutch of gynaecological treatises, most if not all of them translated from the Greek.

In summary, the contents are as follows:

1. Isaac Syri, *Viaticum* 'a Constantino in Latinam linguam translatum' (TK 1298), fols 1-50v
2. *Liber de oblivione* 'a Constantino Africano editus' (TK 1037), fols 51r–v
3. *Constantini Africani de melancholia libri duo* (TK 528), fols 51v–58v

4. *Cleopatrae Arsinoes sororis Gynaecia* (Desideranti tibi filia karissima) (TK 403), fols 58v–60
5. Galen, *De gyneceis*, translated by Nicholas of Reggio (TK 385), fols 60v–62
6. *Ex genitia Muscionis* (Non omnes quidem), preceded by list of contents (TK 922), fols 62–66v

This text, which is such an important source for the Middle English version, has never been published: as the list of contents provides the basis for the chapter numbers used in the Commentary it is transcribed below, with the addition of the chapter numbers and an indication of the corresponding folio numbers.

fols. 62r–v	[1]	Qve mulieres purgantur
fol. 62v	[2]	Quamdiu puelle uirgines esse debeant
	[3]	Que sunt apte ad concipiendum
	[4]	Quid tempus aptius ad concipiendum
	[5]	Quomodo vii mense agant pregnantes
	[6]	Quomodo viii mense
	[7]	Quomodo viiii mense
	[8]	Qve signa aborsus sunt
	[9]	Qve signa proximi partus sint
fols 62v–63r	[10]	Si secunde remanserint
fol. 63r	[11]	Ad lac stringendum
	[12]	Ad feruorem mamillarum
	[13]	Quomodo probatur infans ad nutriendum
	[14]	Qvibus recte nascatur mensibus
	[15]	Qvomodo umbilicus incidatur
	[16]	Quando uel unde infans cibetur
	[17]	Cuius lac accipiat infans
	[18]	Qualis queratur nutrix
	[19]	Ut nutrix salsa non comedat
fols 63r–v	[20]	Ad lac corruptum
fol. 63v	[21]	Quotiens infans in die lactetur
	[22]	Quotiens lactandus sit
	[23]	Quando gestetur
	[24]	Quandiu lactetur
	[25]	Ad profluuium potio
	[26]	Ad disinteriam
	[27]	Ad cursum mulierum mutandum
	[28]	Signa prefocationis matricis et cura
	[29]	Signa ostensionis matricis et cura
fols 63v–64r	[30]	Signa inflationis matricis et cura

fol. 64r	[31]	Signa tumoris matricis et cura
	[32]	Signa duritie matricis et cura
	[33]	Signa doloris matricis post partum et cura
fols 64r– v	[34]	Signa mole id est duritie matricis et cura
fol. 64v	[35]	Signa sanguinationis matricis et cura
	[36]	Signa fluxus sanguinis matricis et cura
	[37]	Signa gonor'r'ee et cura
	[38]	Signa lassitudinis uulue et cura
fols 64v– 65r	[39]	Signa paralisis matricis et cura
fol. 65r	[40]	Unde inpediatur partvs
	[41]	Quot scematibus infantes nascantur
	[42]	Si in capite descendat reliqua parte in latere herente
	[43]	Si pedibus iunctis descendat
	[44]	Si grande caput habuerit
	[45]	Si contra naturam positus fuerit
	[46]	Si manum proferat
	[47]	Si ambas manus proferat
	[48]	Si pedes proferat reliquia parte inclinata
	[49]	Si unum pedem eiecerit
	[50]	Si pedem emiserit cum torta manu supra caput
fols 65r– v	[51]	Si divisos partibus uulue infigat
fol. 65v	[52]	Si caput contortum habuerit
	[53]	Si genua ostendat
	[54]	Si naticas ostendat
	[55]	Si caput et plantas simul ostendat
	[56]	Si diuisus iaceat uel supinus uel indentibus
	[57]	Si plures uno fuerint
fols 65v– 66v	[58]	Ad ulcera et duritiam mamillorum et uermes

7. *Dictionarium Herbarum*

On fol. 67 appears the early Middle English gloss 'Absinthium id est werewod', using the runic character wynn, which went out of use in the thirteenth century. Clearly this is a manuscript that was either written in England or was in England by then.

CHAPTER THREE

Textual Introduction

T he versions in the five extant manuscripts described in the previous chapter differ markedly. The passage considered in the General Introduction on the 'diversities' between men and women (D40–51) illustrates the possible degree of variation, which is of such a nature as to make a conventional critical edition inappropriate. For the classic theory of editing, which attempts to reconstruct an archetype by recension and establishing the genealogical relations between manuscripts through the study of 'common errors', makes a fundamental assumption: that medieval scribes would strive to copy the exemplars in front of them as accurately as possible. This was no doubt the case in certain types of texts, that is, those considered to possess great intrinsic authority, such as the Scriptures, the writings of the Fathers, and classical texts. But it is clear that not all texts were treated with such respect, and this is particularly true of vernacular texts. In a manuscript culture every copy of a text could be, and often was, literally handcrafted for a particular audience: this could entail considerable adaptation, excision, addition, and censorship. So differences in readings, which may be extensive, are not necessarily tell-tale errors at all, but may be deliberate changes that the scribe probably regarded as distinct improvements on his original.

A medical text might merit as careful copying as any other authoritative text, quite apart from the practical need to transmit recipes accurately. But another factor could be at work that would pull in the opposite direction to discourage the automatic, faithful transmission of the exemplar: the nature of the subject matter. *The Knowing of Woman's Kind*, in that it inevitably relates to sexual practices, ventures into territory that can quickly become forbidden. So in the passage in question on sexual difference the vocabularies used by Oxford Bodley MS Douce 37 (Douce) and CUL MS Ii. 6. 33 (Cambridge) diverge sharply. Douce's choice of anatomical terminology, especially for the female genitals, is more detailed, differentiated, and precise than that used by Cambridge (this is demonstrated and discussed further below). This must be a very real consideration in assessing the relative utility, and therefore textual reliability, of these two presumably practical manuscripts. For it is likely that the more nuanced vocabulary is closer to the original wording of the translation, as it would be harder to introduce specificity into a text where the terminology had been originally vague and imprecise than to reverse the process.

Douce is therefore regarded as 'superior' to Cambridge, at least from the narrowly textual point of view, and as the 'best' manuscript, though by no means perfect. But this edition is based on both Douce and Cambridge, as these two manuscripts represent rather different versions of the text, each with its own virtues and characteristics. They are presented on facing pages as the differences between them are such that a critical edition presenting a single text would obscure or destroy a great deal of interesting information that each has to offer. Of the three remaining manuscripts, Oxford Bodley MS 483 is collated with Douce, and BL MS Sloane 421A with Cambridge (only substantive, not orthographical or morphological, variants are given). Selected readings are recorded from BL MS Additional 12195, which is anomalous but closer to Douce than to Cambridge. This too will be considered further below.

Even though two distinct versions of the text are now extant, it can be demonstrated that all the Middle English versions descend from a single Middle English copy. All five share certain 'common errors', readings that can be shown to be indisputably erroneous by reference to the known Latin or French sources. At D284 Douce reads 'oyle ceroine', while Cambridge and Sloane read 'oyle cyroyne'. The only meaning that MED gives for *ciroin* or *ceroin*, a kind of plaster made mainly from wax, is not appropriate here, where the Latin reads 'oleo uiridi'. The erroneous ME readings, though not identical, must derive from a common source; one may speculate that the original reading of the ME was 'oyle ciperine', from the Latin word for henna shrub, and this was then corrupted in the archetype from which all the surviving ME versions ultimately descend.

A clearer and therefore more satisfactory example of a 'common error' is found at DC558 where Douce reads *vrelyon* and Cambridge *vrelion*. The other manuscripts are unanimous in offering spellings with initial *v*, but no such word is recorded by MED. The French source here has *yrilion* and its Latin source, *yrelion*, probably meaning 'a sort of ointment or salve'. It is obvious that an error was made at an early stage of the transmission process and passed on to both textual families. A minor example of the same process, though unsupported by a French or Latin source, can be found at DC580. All the manuscripts here spell their various versions of 'sternutacion' (apparently with the unrecorded sense 'a preparation that causes sneezing') with medial *-m-*, which is obviously wrong. Finally at D872/C871 D reads *affrotitri*, B *a fortigry* and CS *affrotiri*. Clearly there was a problem here at an early stage: the corresponding Latin reads *afronitri,* 'aphronitrum, washing soda', but the Douce and Cambridge family readings almost certainly go back to the same erroneous reading, possibly most closely preserved in Douce's *affrotitri*, which was then further corrupted.

Oxford Bodley MS Douce 37 and Cambridge University Library MS Ii. 6. 33

Douce, at approximately 13,500 words, is about 1500 words longer than Cambridge. Although it includes some additional material, this difference in length is largely attributable to its more expansive style and approach. This is possibly a style adopted for didactic purposes and designed to guide an audience not accustomed to written texts. For instance, Douce provides what are effectively chapter-headings, detailing what it has just discussed and what it plans to discuss next. Thus it reads, 'Now schell I tell yow wyche women may lese her flovrys with-owtyn dysesse' (D113–14), where Cambridge simply states, 'The cause why women lese here flowres ar these' (C113). It prefixes other sections, 'Nov schall I tell yow why þys iij anguysch þat I spake of by-fore fallyn to women rathyre then to men' (D130–31); 'But fyrst I woll tell yow where-of the flouris comme & þan schall I tell yow þe cause of retencyon & defaut & þe cause of superfluyte of hem & þan schall I tell þe medycyn for eche of hem' (D173–76); 'Now schall I tell yow þe cause of retencyon and fayllynge of floures' (D204–05). Where Cambridge reads simply, 'What is the secundyne', Douce has 'And yf ye woll know what ys a secvndyne, I schall tell yow' (D295). A particularly comprehensive example is, 'Now syth I have told yow þe medycyns for superfluite of flourys, now will I tell yow medycyns for þe retencion'

(D663–64), where Cambridge has simply a heading 'Medicines for retencion'.

Further evidence of careful planning can be found in references to material yet to be discussed: for instance, Douce explains the dangers of menstrual failure, unless this is the result of 'þeys cavsys þat I shev here-aftyre' (D108–09), where Cambridge reads simply, 'thes causes her folwynge' (C107). Douce even on occasion provides specific cross-references, as when it mentions 'medycyns þat sewyn here-aftyre, where hit spekyth yf women have to lytyll of here flourys' (D221–22), and 'medycynys þat ye schall fynde here-aftere where hit spekith for superfluite of ouer-moche flovrys' (D245–47). Most elaborate of all, perhaps, is the injunction, 'let euery woman þat trauelyth be welle ware than whan sche hath travelyd þat þe humors þat ys wrytyn on þe nexte syde [i.e. page] comme forth clene' (D867–69), where Cambridge refers merely to 'þat humour that is wreten heer-aftir' (C867).

Douce does also provide some additional information not found in Cambridge. Sometimes this is useful, for instance a digression on skin pores: 'There her lytyll holys full on a mannys body & womannys, not so gret as þe poynt of a nedyll, be the whyche swet got ovte of a man & of a woman & þey been powrys' (D503–05). Douce is also more likely than Cambridge to expand bald statements: so it writes, in reference to menstruation, that women are 'purgyt at her wyket of a mortall poyson þat a-rysyth in hem of a corrupte blode' (D102–03), rather than Cambridge's briefer, but more enigmatic, 'purgyd of corrupcion that risith in hem of corrupte blood' (C101–02); and Douce has 'but lok ye gyve hym not hys modyrs mylk for be-cause of þe travelynge þat sche hath had & þe purgacyon, for þat mylk ys not so good and holsame as oþer' (D470–73), where Cambridge reads 'but not of his mooder firste, be-cause of here traueylynge, for that mylke is not so holsum to hym at the firste as othir woman mylke is' (C470–72). Other minor expansions in the interests of clarity, such as 'þe rote of a herbe þat ys callyd comfyry' (D656) for 'the rote camfory' (C654), or 'þe juse of þe forseyde herbys' (D686–87) for simply 'þe juce' (C687) are common. There are however two cases where Cambridge explains more than Douce, glossing the Latinate 'polipodium' (rather than the Anglicized 'polipodin' found in Douce) with 'that is fern that growith on an ok' (C616), and expanding 'draw hit þorow a cloth' (D699–700) to 'drawe oute the juce therof throw a cloth' (C699–700).

Douce also includes several recipes not found in Cambridge, for instance:

tak þe rote of gladyoll & þe rote of louache & þe herbe of nepte & seth them to-gythyre in wynne & 3if hare to drynk at euyn & at morvnne & let kyuere hare warme þat sche may svete. (D735–38).

Another Douce addition is a charm for a woman in childbirth:

Or tak a lytyll scrowe & wryt þys with-in: + In nomine Patris et Filij & Spiritus Sancti Amen + Sancta Maria + Sancta Margareta + ogor + sugor + nogo + and kyt þat scrov in-to small þecys & 3iffe here to drynk. (D369–72).

But this manuscript is not otherwise more superstitious, perhaps just more traditional in its outlook.

Another reason for Douce's greater length compared to Cambridge is the markedly more personal tone it often adopts. Sometimes it speaks in the first person pronoun; hence it reads:

But sche þat wol haue no travyll in chyldynge, let kepe here fro þe recevynge of sede of man &, oon my parell, sche schall nevyre drede þe travelynge of chylde. (D135–38),

where Cambridge reads tersely, 'Ffor this is no medycyne but kepe fro man' (C134). Douce addresses the reader regularly as *ye* or *yow*, as in 'þe cause þer-of I schall schev yow by resonne. I have tolde yow here be-fore þat þe matryce is made of synow' (D140–42), where Cambridge has simply, 'the cause is this' (C141). Similarly, when describing 'precipitacion or prefocacion' of the womb it reads, 'þe cause of þat payne I schall tel yow' (D155–56) rather than Cambridge's more impersonal 'the cawse ther-of' (C155); it reads, 'But furste y schall wryth my medycyns for delyuerance of chyde' (D359) rather than 'But firste ye shal see mo medicynes for diliueraunce of child' (C359); and 'be-cause þer be many maner of apostemys, both on a man & woman, I will wryt to yow in what maner ye schall know on fro a-noþer' (D1013–15), rather than 'heer may ye knowe how ye shal knowe on fro a-nother' (C1014–15).

In some aspects of its vocabulary Douce contrasts sharply with Cambridge. Its choice of anatomical terms, especially those relating to the genitals, is both more detailed and more specific than those used by Cambridge. Douce writes: 'The iiij diuersite ys by-tvene here leggis, for ... þer hathe women an opynynge wyche ys calde in Frenche a bele chose or ellys a wykket of þe wombe' (D46–49), while Cambridge has: 'The fourte diuersite be-twyn here leggys, for ... ther haue women an openynge callid a cunte or priuyte of the wombe' (C45–48). But after this promising opening Cambridge loses its lexicographical nerve and from then on consistently uses the vague term *priuyte*, while Douce continues to use *wykket* to refer to the female external genitals.

Cambridge generally prefers to refer to the female genitals and reproductive organs in vague terms. While Douce describes the womb as having 'a longe nekk & strayte & large mowthe & a large entre' (D57–58), Cambridge omits the reference to the 'large entre'; Douce describes how, when a woman miscarries, 'a black vrine passyth oþer-wyle at here wyket' (D306–07) while Cambridge confines itself to the comment, 'she makith other-whyle blak vryn' (C306). Elsewhere, Douce describes the need to make sure the child does not 'cleue vn-to þe sydys of þe nek of þe matryce' (D383): in Cambridge the baby merely clings 'to the matrice' (C384). Where Douce explains that hermaphrodites have 'þe tokyn bothe of man & of woman, þat ys bothe yerde and wikket' (D76–77), Cambridge omits the explanatory gloss. Cambridge is generally somewhat squeamish, which seems inappropriate and unhelpful in a gynaecological treatise: when Douce prescribes how a poultice of leeks should be removed once the child is born, 'or ellys all hare bovellys will sew aftyre' (D337–38), Cambridge contents itself with warning, 'for ell all will come after' (C336).

Douce is also more explicit in its references to sexual intercourse. In describing how the woman might conceive a male child, it urges, 'let heere dresse in suche a manere wise here dedyut' (D78–79), while Cambridge is more periphrastic: 'let her dresse here in suche maner wise in the deede of hire naturall lykynge' (C79–80). Later, Douce discusses at what age 'a mayden may vse resonably þe dedyut of dewery' (D249–50), but Cambridge asks, 'At what age a woman may vse hire body naturaly with man' (C249–50). Douce describes how some women 'woll not suffyre hare hosbonde to haw do with hem be way of deduit drwere' (D900–01) while Cambridge simply says, 'they may not suffre naturally with man' (C899–900). Douce consistently uses 'þe deduit' and 'þe deduit of drewery' as terms for sexual intercourse where Cambridge has terms or phrases such as 'the naturall deede' and 'to dele naturally with man'.

Deduit and *drewerie* are both words associated with courtly discourse. Both are borrowed from Old French, and are at home in the romances, for instance. Possibly they were not even understood by some medieval English readers if they were unacquainted with such literature. Substitute phrases employing the native terms *deal* and *deed* may have been used for socio-linguistic rather than stylistic reasons. Is it sheer coincidence that 'the deduit' and 'the dede' look similar? Or that the Douce scribe has so much trouble with his Old French loan words? He often spells *deduit* as *dedyut* or *deuyt*, and *drewerie* as *dewery*, neither of them accepted as a variant spelling by MED, which suggests that the words were unfamiliar to him.

Douce's more explicit language is again evident when, on the subject of sexual activity late in pregnancy, it advises 'þat in þat tyme sche entermet hyre not with no disport of deuyt ... for with suche puttynge þe secundynne myght brek' (D291–93), while Cambridge warns 'that she dispose not here body naturally with man ... ffor with that werke she myght breke the secundyne' (C290–91). Along with this blunter sexual vocabulary goes a more orthodox or rigid moral attitude than that of Cambridge. As some of the examples above illustrate, Douce consistently refers to sexual partners as husbands where Cambridge speaks simply of men, either by implication or explicitly (e.g. D81, 901). And where Douce predicts that a girl who becomes sexually active too early will be 'to lauy of here body to oþer þan to here hosbande' (D256–57) Cambridge simply says, 'she shal be lavy of here body' (C257).

Douce is both fuller and more forthright when it explains how a miscarriage may occur:

summe women vsyn a þynge for they schold not conceyve & þat makyth abortyf, & slen hem-selfe al-so, the whych I dare not wryte lest sume cursyde calet wold hit vse. (D309–11).

In contrast, Cambridge attributes such an event with studious vagueness to 'mysgydynge of her-self' (C308). It also omits Douce's remark, when discussing methods of provoking menstruation, 'Othyre thyngis were good for hare to vse but þat woll not I wryht lest summe wolde leue all þes medycynys & vse þat to moche' (D753–55). This is probably an oblique reference to one popular method of regulating menstruation, that is, by engaging in sexual intercourse, mentioned at this point by the Old French source (along with cupping and scarification, neither of them likely sources of overindulgence). In their different ways both English manuscripts refuse to advocate this practice.

While Douce is likely to be closer than Cambridge to the original Middle English translation, the modifications found in Cambridge are sufficiently interesting, and so thoroughgoing, as to merit its presentation as a version of the text in its own right. On the other hand, the variations are systemic and pervasive, to such an extent that a full and accurate collation would be almost impossible to carry out and would also make the complete text of Cambridge hard for the modern reader to reconstruct. Hence the decision to present the two texts side by side.

Oxford MS Bodley 483

MS Bodley 483 is closely related to Douce, with which it shares a common source. It is a 'good' manuscript that occasionally is the only one out of all five with a reading that makes sense. For instance, after a passage detailing two magic charms, Douce reads: 'But wethyth well þat þis ne nonne oþer kepyth no woman at commenabyll tyme of delyuerance & þer-for let þe mydwyffe helpe' (D374–76). Cambridge and Sloane say much the same (C371–73), which suggests the reading might be original, but it seems strange for this text to repudiate so abruptly something it had just taken the trouble to describe in detail. But Bodley adds, 'but as a preparatyue', immediately before '& þer-for let þe mydwyffe helpe'. It also provides some phrases omitted by Douce (e.g. D116–17, 321–22, D682–83) that must have been present in their common source: this demonstrates that Bodley is not derived from Douce. And it also provides a number of individual readings that are sometimes better (that is, more obviously correct) than those of Douce (e.g. D198, 507). It has therefore been used from time to time to correct Douce when Douce's reading was clearly unsustainable or defective.

Bodley also seems to have tried hard to make sense of the text where there were problems, though not always successfully. For instance, at D912–13 Douce reads, 'And yf þe payne lest, tak kycumbres'. It is clear from the Latin here ('Si paruus sit dolor') that *laste*, the reading of CS, is wrong, as is D's if *lest* is a form of *last*. The original reading must have been *lesse*, 'lessen, grow less'. Bodley seems to have felt uncomfortable with the ambiguity of the reading, but went for the wrong solution, by supplementing *lest* with 'lest longe'.

Like all the versions, Bodley provides its own occasional glosses. At D293 it adds to *secundynne* the phrase 'or skynne' (even though the text goes on to give a detailed explanation of 'what ys a secvndyne'), while at D860 where the text describes how, if one strikes the swollen uterus, 'hit will sond as hit were a tabure', B reads (somewhat fancifully) 'a belle or a tabure'.

But any claims that Bodley might have had to be used as a base text are undermined by its choice of gynaecological vocabulary. It is the one manuscript that flatly refuses, in its description of the 'fourth diversity' between men and women, to give any sort of name to the female genitals. Later in the text it is not surprising that the use of some term becomes unavoidable, but Bodley consistently refuses to use *wikket*. Unlike Cambridge (and Sloane, see further below), however, it never uses *pryuete*, instead using the periphrastic phrase 'mowthe' (or occasionally, e.g. D290, *entre*) 'of her/the wombe'. There are numerous examples of this phrase (e.g. D537, 562, 568, etc.). This solution is ambiguous at best and when on occasion Bodley uses *wombe* alone (e.g. D935) could also be misleading. It could even be dangerous when, for instance, Douce refers to the need to avoid the baby catching its feet on the 'sydys of þe wyket' as it is born (D350), Bodley substitutes 'syde of þe mouthe of the wombe'. Bodley is also prepared to change the meaning in order to avoid *wikket*: at D74 where Douce refers to corruptions that pass 'ovt by þe wyket', Bodley reads 'vp from the wombe', which surely means something quite different. Only on one occasion does Bodley preserve *wekett*, which suggests that its exemplar did use the term (in which it was followed by Douce) and that the redactor of Bodley was deliberately following a 'global replace' procedure which was not infallible.

Bodley, like Cambridge, also dislikes the terms *dedyut* or 'dedyut of drewery' and resorts to various constructions to avoid them. It substitutes 'resonable vse to dele with man' for 'vse resonably þe dedyut of dewery' (D249–50); 'sche entermet not of dedeuyt of dewery' becomes 'she entermet hyr not with man' (D483–84); and *dedyut* becomes 'to dele with man' (D253). But its substitution of 'to deale with her by the way of deduit' for Douce's 'tuche here be-twex þe deduit' (D934) suggests that if *deduit* was too explicit, *tuche* was even worse.

Finally, Bodley almost imperceptibly distances itself from its subject matter. When listing the three complaints 'þat principally dysesyn women' (D86–87), it substitutes *them* for *women*, and later in discussing failure of the flowers, 'as whanne a woman hath nonne' (D665), it substitutes *þei* for 'a woman'. This is perhaps connected with the fact that Oxford MS Bodley 483 is a compendium of general medical texts, only some of which are concerned with women's health, and may well have been compiled for a male reader.

British Library MS Sloane 421A and MS Additional 12195

These two manuscripts have virtually no significant textual value in the narrow sense of contributing to the recovery of an archetype or constructing a 'critical edition'. But they are valuable from other points of view. Consequently, substantive readings from MS Sloane are fully recorded, while readings from MS Additional are given selectively, for reasons that will become clear.

The text found in BL MS Sloane 421A is in general an inferior, more careless, version of CUL MS Ii. 6. 33, containing hardly any independent readings of value. In other words in traditional terms it is a 'bad manuscript'. But every medieval manuscript gives a version of a text that was created for particular reasons, for a particular audience, although only too often we can now perceive these but dimly. The Sloane manuscript is a case in point: it has a real interest if one's concern is with the transmission and reception, rather than reconstruction, of this text. It claims to have been translated, or adapted, not just for the benefit of women in general but at the request of a specific woman. When the redactor and/or scribe writes, 'after the treatys of dyuers masters ... I haue drawen & wrytten in Inglishe & at the pleasure of my ladye' (cf. C22–23), the final phrase, '& at the pleasure of my ladye', is unique to his version of the text.

Sloane is about 500 words shorter than Cambridge, its closest textual relative, and often seems adapted to censor or tone down even further some of the more unpalatable or alarming aspects of childbirth and sex. In a description of the newly delivered mother who, according to Cambridge, 'lyth otherwhile as ded, but that hire yes be not turned vpward' (C907–08), Sloane just has 'so that she lyethe otherwhile as deid'. In a section on 'slackness of the privity', an affliction resulting in a woman's reluctance to have sexual relations, the consequences if she is forced to do so are spelt out by Cambridge:

> yif it [the seed of man] abyde and conceyue it shal be [abhors], so that the child shal the secunde monyth or the thirde be formyd, but it shal be slendir and litill. (C978–80).

Sloane completely omits this, even at the cost of ruining the sense.

Typically, then, Sloane omits material. By luck or good judgement, it omits two of the more superstitious (or traditional) passages. Both are concerned with cures to staunch a woman's bleeding, the one by tying one of her hairs around a tree (C650–52), the other by hanging a bag full of burnt toad around a patient's neck (C636–41). Sloane does include this latter recipe, but the other manuscripts go on to strain our credulity even further by outlining an experiment to prove its efficacy. Hang such a bag around a chicken's neck, decapitate it in two days' time, and it will not bleed. Sloane is wise enough to leave well alone. Another place where it shows good sense in omitting material is in the account of feeding newborn babies. It omits the casual remark, preserved in all the other manuscripts, and probably a misunderstanding of the corresponding Latin (see Commentary), that 'summe men sey that it were good for a child to sowke mylke of ix women

afore his moodris mylk and aftir þat his moodris mylke is beste to hym'
(C473–76).

But Sloane does sometimes expand. It is, for instance, the only manuscript
to gloss 'precipitation of þe matrice' as *dyslocacyon* (note to C88). Perhaps
precipitation was a technical term that the redactor knew his reader would
find unfamiliar: in fact, neither MED nor OED record the medical meaning
of prolapse that is appropriate here. And in one recipe the ingredient *muste*
(C557) is, literally, glossed above the line as 'i.e. vinygre'. Another more
extensive expansion, unique to Sloane, occurs in the description of one type
of malpresentation, when 'the child lyth a-yens kende' (C391): Sloane adds,
'that is when he commethe furthe hes face loking vp to hes mothers face'.
Perhaps the redactor regarded the original description as too vague for an
inexperienced reader, or perhaps he wanted to demystify the idea of the
'unnatural'. Finally, when the treatise, in all its versions, inveighs against
those who feed a failing wet-nurse with *estreen* of sheep or cow, which
'encombrith here stomak that she may not defie her mete and so turnyth to
corrupcion and hurtith the child' (C488–90), Sloane amplifies this by adding,
'and so the nvrse have no mylke', spelling out the reasons for caution,
obvious though they may be.

This tendency towards explication is linked with a similar impulse
towards simplification and familiarization. Sloane simplifies a somewhat
exotic recipe, 'make her a pissarye of vrelion, mostelion, camelys, nardileo,
for thes wil drawe the sedis and the floures down' (C557–59), to 'make her a
pissarye of the same [i.e. lignum aloe, musk and vinegar] with woll'. It
reduces the impressive list of laxatives, 'trifera serracyneise, ebrose, sirep of
violet and other suche laxatifiis' (C613–14), to *laxatyue*s pure and simple. It
omits altogether a recipe for a *stermutacion* (C580–82), something to make
the patient sneeze, perhaps as too obscure. And its substitution of
swadbondis (swaddling clothes) for the reading of all other manuscripts,
wymplis (C955), may also be part of a desire to be more comprehensible to a
lay audience, unless it reflects that audience's relatively low social status.

Some of these simplifications may be due to the redactor and/or scribe's
own lack of expertise rather than that of his audience, for Sloane betrays a
certain confusion over terminology from time to time. It writes for instance
of 'the emerodis or the fire' rather than, more correctly, 'emerawdys' or 'the
ffy' (C769) where *ffy* translates the Latin *ficus* (piles, haemorrhoids),
although this meaning is not recorded in MED. In one recipe it lists
astrologye as an ingredient in a medical recipe instead of *aristologe*
(birthwort) (C788), and it corrupts 'braunchis of vrsyn' (C1051) (bear's

breech or acanthus), to 'branches of vyne'. The text is similarly uneasy with
medical authorities: it refers to a pessary as used by 'dame fabiane prynces'
where Cambridge has 'Dame Ffabyan Prycelle' (C719–20), a lady whose
name is directly borrowed from the Old French source. And although it
includes a recipe introduced in Cambridge as 'Anodir medycyn that a lady
Salerne vsid' (C685), it does not give the attribution.

Finally, its gynaecological vocabulary is reticent, even more so than that
of Cambridge. In the section discussing the physiological differences
between men and women Sloane, after a detailed account of the first three
diversities, writes laconically, 'The fourthe is of ther preue members', where
the other four manuscripts describe and name (admittedly in their own ways)
the male and female genitals (C46–48). Elsewhere when it is unavoidable,
Sloane like Cambridge consistently uses the euphemistic, and unhelpful,
phrase 'previte of the wombe' for the external female genitals, rather than
Douce's anatomically precise *wykket*. Possibly this provides further evidence
that this version was indeed made for a particular woman, who may have
been young and relatively inexperienced in such matters (recently married,
perhaps, and expecting her first child). But it is unfortunate that we know
absolutely nothing about the original ownership of this manuscript, and so
cannot speculate further about the woman for whom this version of the text
was created.

As we have seen, there is in fact only one manuscript about which we
have any information as to provenance. BL MS Additional 12195 offers a
severely abbreviated version of the text, a good 2000 words shorter than
Douce, to which it is somewhat distantly allied. Like Sloane, there is some
evidence that this version was made for a particular woman. It is arguable
that there appears to be a parenthetical address to 'my ladye' in the section
on different types of apostemes or swellings, where none of the other
manuscripts have any equivalent phrase: 'The iiij comythe of fleme & is
called zymia and thes apostemys, my ladye, schall ye knowe be þes signes'
(cf. D1020). Unfortunately the reading is not indisputable; the final letter is
probably *e* but as final *e* and final *s* are hard to distinguish in this hand the
reading here might be *myladys*, presumably a corruption of *maladys*, in
apposition to *apostemys*. Or it might even be *myladyo*, as final *e* and final *o*
are also similar, though in this case it would be impossible to say what was
meant.

Even more so than Sloane, Additional badly garbles technical terms,
which suggests that the scribe and/or adapter was not accustomed to medical
or gynaecological texts. For instance, A reads *garagodion* for *geralogodion*

or *yeralogadyon* (D616); *langao* for *longaon* (D157); *emerowndys* for *emeroydys* (D217); *horsnes* or *hors* for *abhors* (D864, 951); 'jmpensethy onnenus' for 'herpesethi omenus' (D1018–19); and 'ffera magna' for 'trifera magna' (D775). Other obscure terms it simply omits.

As its relative length suggests, Additional has several extensive cuts, though we cannot know how far this is deliberate and how far the result of a defective exemplar. A lengthy omission of about 300 words occurs in a section that covers the choice and management of the wet-nurse, discerning which children will be 'esy to norsche', and infant care during the first year of life and weaning. This is all material that goes back to Soranus's *Gynaecia* and it constitutes just about the sum total of the treatise's advice on childcare. In another section Additional omits a medicinal drink of the common herb horehound and wine, a bath of horehound, a poultice of horehound, and subfumigation with horehound (D699–706). (Elsewhere it substitutes *fume* for *suffumigacion*, a term it uses only once and a practice in which it seems to have little faith.) Another series of four remedies that it omits are for a poultice of colrage and radish, for the bark of the cherry tree, a third drawn from *Ypocras*, that is, Hippocrates, and a fourth recommendation that the patient should eat anything she fancies (D763–73). Perhaps the passage contained too many unfamiliar technical terms. Further omissions include the symptoms of paralysis of the uterus (D984–91), and about 200 words describing recipes to 'ripen' different types of apostemes classified by the humours. Curiously, these omissions are not evenly distributed throughout the treatise but become more extensive as it progresses, almost as if the redactor were becoming increasingly critical or impatient with the text (or texts) before him.

When it does not omit it may radically simplify and condense. For instance, in the Prologue it reads succinctly: 'And therfor every woman redet vn to oþer þat can not so do and helpe hem & concell theme in her maladis with owt schewyng her desses vnto man.' Douce has a longer, more convoluted explanation:

> And be-cause whomen of our tonge cvnne bettyre rede & vndyrstande þys langage þan eny other and euery whoman lettyrde rede hit to oþer vnlettyrd & help hem & conceyle hem in here maledyes with-owtyn schevynge here dysese to man, I have þys drawyn & wryttyn in Englysch. (D18–22).

Consequently Additional does not labour the point about women's ignorance of Latin (and also, it is implied in Sloane, of French) or even make much of the illiteracy of some women in English. Nor does it parade the claim that the text's sources are by 'dyuerse mastrys þat have translatyde hem oute of

Grek in-to Latyn' (D17–18). It also considerably simplifies the numerous
herbal remedies. For instance, out of a paragraph that recommends in turn a
barley and plantain tisane, bean water, a poultice of wheat, honey, and milk,
and a plaster of sheep's dung or chicken grease (D625–31), it keeps only one
recommendation: 'it is good for here to drunke þe water þat benys is sothen
in.'

Sometimes however it simplifies at the cost of changing the meaning.
Where Douce reads:

> And yf hit so be þat a woman have not hem [menstrual periods] euery monyth
> onys fro þe tyme sche [may] [conceyve], þat ys fro xv yere, till sche be fyfty
> wyntyr olde, ... sche schall sodenly dey (D106–12),

Additional substitutes a much less alarming, and more positive, statement,
'þo women þat have þeme every monyth onys, þei may conceyve fro xv yere
tyll þei be l wynter olde'. For this version has a mind of its own and makes
some entirely original contributions to the text. In the discussion of how to
cut the umbilical cord, Additional is unique in suggesting 'a peyere of sheris'
rather than 'a sharpe knyffe' (D459–60). It also omits the censure of old
wives' practices in this respect as witchcraft (D460–63), which as we have
seen can be traced right back to Soranus. And the final half-page which
replaces the last two pages of Douce is unique to this manuscript. It
comprises a medicine to 'put the uterus into its right place', a description of
the dangers of honey, fennel, and cumin for a pregnant woman, and a
prescription to shrink a woman's stomach.

Textually, this version belongs to the same family as Douce and Bodley,
rather than Cambridge and Sloane, but surprisingly it does sometimes follow
the latter in minor details. Even more puzzling, it occasionally gives readings
from both families, as alternatives. For instance, it reads 'mire or of a nutre'
where D reads *myrre* (D729) and C reads *nutre* (C729); and 'modirwort or
mogwode' where D reads *mvgwort* (D831) and C reads *moodir-wort* (C830).

Further evidence that this version of the text might have been deliberately
made more accessible to women is its comment on childbirth, 'þat caus
every whoman knowyth', rather than Douce's 'euery body knovth' (D90) or
Cambridge's 'euery discreet body knowith' (C90–91), or its gloss on the
vessels of the uterus (D67) as 'ye chamberes or vesselus'. Its gynaecological
terminology is plain and decent: it follows Douce in naming the female
genitals as an 'opynynge weche is called a bel chos or ells a weket of the
wombe' (cf. D48–49), but it omits the phrase 'in Frenche' after 'a bel chos',
which again might suggest a desire to avoid an unnecessary parade of

learning. From then on it is the only manuscript to follow Douce in consistently using *weket* where appropriate.

It is tempting to suggest that the redactor, as well as the designated reader, of this version might have been a woman. The simplifications, omissions, and misunderstandings; the avoidance of an undue appearance of learning; and the occasional woman-friendly remark: all could be adduced to support this view. Moreover, the text itself, though written out competently enough, contains many spellings that are unconventional, even by ME standards: for instance, such contractions as *havit* for 'have it', or *redyt* for 'reade yt', and so on. This possibility would not necessarily be precluded by the evidence, already discussed, that the manuscript of which this text is part may have belonged to a house of Augustinian canons in North Creake, Norfolk.

A further feature of interest is the extensive rubrication of this particular copy. This suggests that, even if not owned by or written for a woman, it might have been designed to be made available for consultation by those known to be relatively inexperienced with books. Medieval texts can be hard to navigate: for instance it may not even be clear where one text ends and another begins, and chapter headings and lists of contents are often not provided, let alone titles. But Additional would present few problems as long as one could read, as it highlights new topics and key terms with the generous use of red ink. Moreover, this is the only manuscript to give the text a contemporary title, *The Knowing of Woman's Kind in Childing*, which has been adopted for this edition. In short, both textually and physically this sets out to be a user-friendly version of the text, even though it omits some useful material and garbles many technical terms.

Because of its extensive and considerable deviations from all the other manuscripts, it has not been practicable to present full collations from Additional. But some substantive readings are recorded, particularly when they support Douce against Bodley, or *vice versa*, or when they are intrinsically interesting. Additional certainly deserves to be studied in its own right as a distinctive version of our text with its own distinctive virtues; and it has in fact been transcribed as part of a University of York MA thesis by Lisa Howarth.

Editorial Procedure

Abbreviations have been expanded conventionally and silently, except for '&' and '3' (symbol for *uncia*, ounce) which are preserved. The letters yogh and thorn have been preserved. Punctuation, capitalization, and paragraphing have all been modernized. The manuscripts' word division has been preserved but lexical units are indicated by the addition of hyphens where necessary. Any emendation to the base text, whether imported from another manuscript or (occasionally) conjectural, is marked with square brackets. Interlinear or marginal additions in the manuscripts are indicated by `' and further information is given in the textual apparatus.

In the extracts from unedited Latin and French texts quoted in the Commentary, abbreviations have again been expanded silently and conventionally. Letters or syllables to be omitted are marked with < >. No systematic attempt has been made to emend these texts, unless the reading the ME translator had before him seems fairly obvious. Such emendations are marked by square brackets and the manuscript reading is also given.

The Texts

Douce Version

[O]vre lorde God, whan he had storid þe worlde, of all creaturis he
made manne & woman resonabull creature and badde hem wexe
and multiply, & ordende þat of þem ij schulde cume þe thurde &
þat of þe man, þat is made of hote & dry mature, schulde come þe
5   sede & þat þe woman, þat ys made of cold matyre & moyste,
schulde receyue þe sede, so þat [be] þe tempure of hote & colde,
moyste & dry, þe chylde schulde be engendyrde, ryht as we seen
treys, cornys & herbys mov not growe with-ovte resonabyll
tempure of þe iiij. And for as moche as whomen ben more febull
10   & colde be nature þan men been & have grete travell in
chyldynge, þer fall oftyn to hem mo diuerse sykenes than to men,
and namly to þe membrys þat ben longyng to gendrynge.
      Wherfore in þe worschyp of oure Lady & of all sayntys I
thynke to do myn ententyffe bysynes for-to drav [f. 1v] oute of
15   Latyn in-to Englysch dyuerse causis of here maladyes, the synes

2 woman] A, + & D, + a B   3 þem ij] j B   4 mature] BD, nature A   5 cold …
moyste] colde & moyst mater B   matyre] D, nater A   6 be] *om.* D, by B   þe …
colde] by temperaunce of colde & hote B   7 ryht] like B   9 tempure] temperaunce B
þe] these B   10 be] of B   11 sykenes] sykenesses B   12 gendrynge] engenderyng BA
13 þe] *om.* BA   14–15 drav … Englysch] schew after the french & latyn þe A

Cambridge Version

Owre lord God, whan he had storid the [world], of all creatures he
made man and woman resonabill creatures and bad hem waxe and
multiplie. And that man, that is hote and drye matier, shuld sowe
the seed, and that the woman, that is made of cold nature and
5 moyste, shuld resseyue the seed, so that be the [tempure] of colde
and hete, moyste and drye, the childe shuld be engendrid, right as
we se trees, cornis and erbis may not growe with-owte tempure of
the foure. And for as meche as women ar more febill and cold be
nature than men and haue gret trauayle in childynge, ther fallith
10 onto them mo diuers syknes than to men, and namely to the
membris [that] longe to engendure.

    Wherfore in the worship of oure Lady and all holy seyntis I
thynke to do myn ententif besynesse to drawe owte [f. 1v] of
15 Frensh and Latyn in-to Inglysh the diuers causes of here maledies,

---

1 world] S, word C   4 the²] *om.* S   made] *om.* S   5 tempure] temperure C,
tempreture S   6 hete] hote S   right] + so S   7 cornis] corne S   8 foure] erthe S
be] of S   11 that] þat S, 'tho' to C   engendure] engendring S   15 Frensh and] *om.* S

þat þey schall knov hem by & þe curys helpynge to hem, afture þe
tretys of dyuerse mastrys þat have translatyde hem oute of Grek
in-to Latyn. And be-cause whomen of oure tonge cvnne bettyre
rede & vndyrstande þys langage þan eny oþer & euery whoman
20 lettyrde [may] rede hit to oþer vnlettyrd & help hem & conceyle
hem in here maledyes with-owtyn schevynge here dysese to man,
I have þys drawyn & wryttyn in Englysch.

And yf hit fall any man to rede hit, I pray hym & scharge hym
25 in ovre Lady be-halue þat he rede hit not in no dyspyte ne
sclavndure of no woman ne for no cause but for þe hele & helpe
of hem, dredynge þat vengavns myht fall to hym as hit hath do to
oþer þat have schevyd here preuytees in sclavndyr of hem,
vndyrstondynge in certeyne þat þey have no oþer euylys þat nov
30 be [f. 2] a-lyue than thoo women hade þat nov be seyntys in
hevyn.
[R]yht as þe makere of all þyngys ordende treys for-to bvrione
& floure & þan aftyrwarde for-to beere froyte, in þe same manere
he hath orde'y'nde to all whomen an esporgymente the whyche ys
35 calde þe flourys, wit-outyn whyche may no chylde be engendryde
ne conceyvyde. For be-foore þat hit ys comyn ne afture hit ys
gonne may no woman conceyue. For ryht as polucyon be
superhabundance of humors fallyth to a man, so dothe þe flovrys
to a woman, as I schall tell yow herc-aftyre.
40 But furste ye schall undyrstonde þat þer be v dyuersyteys
be-tven man & woman. The fyrste dyuersyte ys a-bove here
fronte, for þer be summe men ballyd & so be not women but
seldyn. The ij dyuersyte ys on here berde, for þer be men thyke
heryde & þer be women [f. 2v] smoth. The iij diuersite ys on here

---

16 afture] For this is B   18 be-cause] + that B   19 &²] + þat B   20 may] B, *om.* D
22 þys drawyn] *tr.* B   wryttyn] + it B   Englysch] + tonge B   24 fall] happen B
26 sclavndure] in slawnder B   hele] helpe B   helpe] helþe B   27 dredynge]
+ lesse B   28 have] haþe B   29 vndyrstondynge in certeyne] lattyng you certaynly
know B   29–30 þey … a-lyue] women now alyve have noon oþer evyll B
34 esporgymente] purgacion B, sporgement A   35 þe] *om.* BA   engendryde] born B
36 be-foore] + þe tyme   afture] + þat   37–38 be … man] cometh of
superhabundaunce of humours B   38–39 so … woman] so comyth the flowrys of
woman B   42 fronte] forhede B   43 here] + the here of the B

the signe that ye shal know hem by and the cures helpynge to
them, aftir the tretys of diuers maistris that han translatid owte of
Greek in-to Latyn and Frensh. And be-cawse that women of oure
tunge cunne bettir reede and vnderstonde this langage than ony
20 other, and euery woman lettrid [maye] reede it to other vnlettrid
[and] helpe hem and counseyle hem in here maladyes with-owte
shewynge here dishese to man, I haue this drawen and wreten it in
Inglish.
  And yif it falle any man to reede it, I praye hym and charge
25 hym on oure Lady be-half that he reede it in no despite and
slaundir of no woman nor for no cause but for the hele and helpe
of hem, dredynge that vengeaunce myght falle to hym as it hath
doon to [f. 2] other that hath shewid here prevites in slawndrynge
of hem, vnderstondynge in certeyn that they haue non othir
30 evillys, women that now be on lyve, than tho women had that now
be seyntis in heuene.
  Ffor right as God hath ordeyned trees for-to burion and floure
and aftir-ward to bere frute, in the same maner he hath ordeyned
to all women to haue espurgement callid the floures, with-owte
35 the which may no chyld be conceyuyd a-fore that it is comyn, nor
after that it is gon. Ffor right as pollucion be superhabundaunce of
humours fallyth to a man, so doth the flouris to a woman, as ye
shall see hire-aftir.

40   But firste ye shal vnderstande v diuersites be-twen man and
woman. The firste diuersite is a-boue here fronte, for ther are
summe men ballyd and so ar no women. [The] secunde diuersite
on her berd, for ther ar men þik [f. 2v] herid and women smothe.
The thirde diuersite on her brestis, for ther haue men litill wertis

16 signe] singnes S   17–18 that ... Frensh] *om.* S   18 be-cawse] *om.* S   18–20 of ...
woman] *om.* S   20 maye] S, *om.* C   it] *om.* S   vnlettrid] vnlernyd S   21 and'] S,
an C   22 dishese] dyseases S   this] *om.* S   23 Inglish] + & at the pleasure of my
ladye S   24 falle] happen S   praye hym and] *om.* S   26 hele] helpe S   helpe]
hele S   27 myght] maye S   hym] them S   28 other] others S   29 hem] other S
29–31 vnderstondynge ... heuene] *om.* S   32 hath] *om.* S   for-to ... floure] to burione
flouris S   34 espurgement] esporgementis S   35 that it] the flouris S   36 pollucion]
pollucyons S   40 be-twen] *twice* S   42 The] S, Te C

45 brestys, for þer hath men but lytyll vertis & þer hath women long
    pappis & hangynge. The iiij diuersite ys by-tvene here leggis, for
    þer have men a yerde with oþer portynavns & þer hathe women an
    opynynge wyche ys calde in Frenche a bele chose or ellys a
    wykket of þe wombe. The v dyuersite is þat in þe body of þe
50 woman be-tvene here navyll & here wyket, for þer hath sche a
    vessyll þat no man hath, þe wych ys callyde þe maryce.
        And be-cause hit ys with-in þe woman, þat no man may se what
    hit ys, reson wolde þat I schulde telle yow fyrst how hit ys
    schapyn & [made] & where-of hit is formyde. The matrice ys a
55 vessell made of thyn leddyr, rowgh with-in & playn with-owt &
    slydynge, thykly fretyde & enterlacyde with small synovys all
    a-bovt & hath a longe nekk & strayte & [a] large mowthe & a
    large entre & a plenere euyn schapp [f. 3] lyck [an] vrinall, þe
    bottvm þer-of to þe navyll of þe woman & þe ij sydys to þe ij
60 sydys of þe woman, & hit ys partyde in-to vij vesellys, of þe
    wyche iij lyth in þe party tovarde þe ryȝht syde, & iij in þe party
    tovarde þe lyfte syde, & þe vij evyn in þe myddys be-tvene þe
    navyll & þe wykket. The whyche matrice ys ordende to receyve &
    holde þe sede of man & þe chylde to conceyue, forme & norsche
65 vn-to conuenabyll tyme of hys byrth. And so hit ys rowgh
    with-ynne for-to hold þe sede þat hit goyth not ovte & peryche.
        And yf hit so be þat þe sede fall in-to eny of þe chambyrs of þe
    ryȝht syde, hit schall be a man chyldc yf it þer-in a-byde & be
    conceyvydde, & yf hit falle in-to eny of þe vesels of þe lyfte syde,
70 hit schall be a maydyn schyld, and yf hit fall in-to þe vesyll þat ys
    in þe myddes, hit fallyth owt & [peryschyth] fro þe place of
    creacyon. And yf hit [f. 3v] a-byde hit fallith to corrupcion of þe
    superfluite of hote, cold, drynesse & moysture & oþer corrupcions
    þat passun ovt by þe wyket with-ovtyn resistens to þe sede &
75 rotyth hyt; & yf hit so be-fall þat hit be conceyuyde þer, hit schall

46 by-tvene] be twix B   48 in … chose] ye knowe the name B   in Frenche] *om.* A
48–49 a² … þe] her B   49–50 in … woman] within her body B   50 wyket] wombe
51 maryce] matrice B   54 made] BA, formyde D   57 a²] B, *om.* D   58 a … schapp]
playne and even shapen B, playn schapyn A   an] BA, & D   61 in² … party] *om.* D
63 wykket] wombe B   64 norsche] ther to be noryshed B   67 of²] on B   69 þe¹]
+ iij B   71 peryschyth] perysch D, peryshyth B   73 hote] hete & B   74 ovt …
wyket] vp from the wombe B

45 and women longe pappis and hangynge. The fourte diuersite
be-twyn here leggys, for ther haue men a membir callid a pyntyll
with othir portenaunce and ther haue women an openynge callid a
cunte or priuyte of the wombe. The fyfte diuersite is with-jnne the
body of the woman be-twen her navyl and here pryuyte, for ther
50 she hath a vessell that no man hath, the which is callid the matrice.

   This vessel callid the matrice is a thenne skyn, rowh with-inne
and pleyn with-owte, sclydynge, thikly frettid and enterlasyd with
smale senues all a-bowte, and hath a longe nekke & streyte and a
55 large mowth and plener shapen lyke an vrynall, the botom lyinge
to the navyll of the woman and sydys [f. 3] to sydes of 'þe'
woman, and it is partid in-to vij vessellis, of the which iij ar in the
parte toward the right syde, and iij are in the parte toward the lyfte
syde, and the vij euen in the myddes be-twen the navill and hire
60 pryvite. The which matrice is ordeyned to reseyue and holde the
seed of man, the child to be conseyued, fourmed and norished to
conabill tyme of his birthe.

65

   And yif it so be that the seed falle in-to ony of the chambris of
the ryght syde, it shal be a man childe. And yif it falle in-to ony of
'þe' vessellis of the lyfte syde, it shal be a woman chylde. And if it
70 falle in the myd vessell, it fallith owte a-yen, and perysshith fro
the place of creacion. And if it a-byde it fallith to corrupcion of
the superfluite of hete, colde, drynesse and moystour, and other
[f. 3v] corrupcions that passith vp fro here priuite with-oute
resistence to the seed and rote it. And yif the seed happen ther to
75 be conceyuyd, it shal haue the token both of man and woman, as it

44–45 men ... hangynge] women longe pappes & hangynge & men haue wartis S
45 diuersite] *om.* S   46–48 be-twyn ... wombe] is of ther preue members S   48 is]
om. S   49 body ... woman] womans bodye S   55 botom] + lyke C   57 it] *om.* S
59 myddes] myddill S   the³] her S   hire] the S   60–61 and ... man] the seed of
man to hold S   62 conabill] convenyent S   his] her S   67 it] *om.* S   72 superfluite]
superfluites S   73 passith] goothe S   vp] furthe S   74 to¹] to S   75 token] marke S
of] + the S

have þe tokyn bothe of man & of woman, þat ys bothe yerde and wikket, as hit hath be seynne heere be-fore in many cuntreys.

And þerfor a woman þat wolde conceyue a man childe, let heere dresse in suche a manere wise here dedyut þat here lefte
80 hyppe ly more herere than here ryȝht, for so schall sche make þe seede of here hosbonde to fall on here ryȝht syde where þat þe man ys conceyvydde. And in þe contrarij maner workyth for þe femall.

Nov have I told yow what is þe matryce & how hit lyes in
85 womans body. And nov I wol tell yow þe anguysch þat dysesyth hit: ye schall know fyrst þat þer been iij anguysch þat principally dysesyn women [f. 4] be here marys. The fyrst ys travelynge of chylde. The ij ys suffocacyon, precipitacion or prefocacion of þe marys. The iij ys retencion, defaute or superfluite of flovrys.

90 [T]he fyrst, þat ys chyldynge, euery body knovth. Suffocacion of þe maryce ys an angvych þat doth women to suell at þe poynt of here herte & makyth hem to sovnde & to fall dovne, þer tethe yonyde to-gedyre with-owt dravynge ore schevynge of breth, & but they be holpe þe sonere in suche case hit ys wondure & euere
95 they releve. Prefocacyon or precipytacion of marys make womanys backys vpwarde & donvarde to here [raynys] for-to 'h'ak & makyth here hede for-to hak & all for defautt of resonabull delyuerance of her body, as [ye] schall here heere hereafture.

100 The flourys of women ys anguysch þat fallyth to euery woman be nature euery monyth onys, and at a certayn [tyme] be þey purgyt at [f. 4v] her wyket of a mortall poyson þat a-rysyth in hem of a corrupte blode, so that svmme women have hit euery mon'y'the many dayes and summe women but few dayes, but þey

76 þe] a B   79 a] *om.* B   manere] maner of   80 ly] be B   herere] vp B   ryȝht]
+ hyppe B   81 here²] the B   83 femall] femynyn B   84 in] + a B   85 anguysch]
angwysshes B   85–86 þat … anguysch] *om.* B   87 women] them B   marys]
matrice B   90 þat] *om.* B   chyldynge] + þat ys B   91 maryce] matrice B   92 here]
the B   sovnde] swoone BA   93 ore schevynge] *om.* BA   95 marys] matrice B   96
raynys] ranys D, reynes B   for-to] sore B   98 ye] BA, sche D   here] see B   heere]
om. B   100 women ys] womennys B   101 tyme] BA, *om.* D   101–02 be² … purgyt]
purgyth D, puorget A, they been purged B   102 wyket] wombe B

hath ben se in many cuntres.

    [An] experiment for 'a' woman that will conceyue a man chyld:
let her dresse here in suche maner wise in the deede of hire
80 naturall lykynge: let hire lefte hype lye hier than here right, for so
she shal make the seed of man to falle on the right syde where the
male is conceyued. And in the same maner do on the tother syde
for the female.
    Heer is taught yow what is þe matrice and how it lyth. Now
85 vnderstonde the [syknesses] that deshese it. Ffirst ye shal knowe
that iij syknesses pryncipally dishese women be here matrice. The
firste is traueylyng of child; the secunde is [suffocacyon],
prefo[f. 4]cacion, precipitation of þe matrice. The thirde is
retencioun, defaute [or] superfluite of flours.
90   The firste [is] childynge; that cause euery discreet body
knowith. Suffocacion of the matrice is a syknesse that makith a
woman to swelle at the poynte of here herte [& cawsethe her] to
swone and to falle down, hire teeth [joyned] to-gedir with
shewyng of breth, and but they be holpe in suche cas it is wonder
95 yif they leue. Prefocacion or precipitacion of the matrice makith
her backys vpward and downward to the reynes for-to ake, and hir
hed for-to ake, al for deliueraunce of hire body, as ye shal see
aftirward.

100   The flowris is a syknes that fallith to euery woman be nature
euery monyth onys at a certeyn tyme, and than are they purgyd of
corrupcion that risith in hem of corrupte blood, so that summe
women haue it many dayes [f. 4v] and sume but fewe dayes,
summe surfetously and summe lytill while and esyly. This

78 An] And C, Ane S   80 hire] + lift her S   here] the S   81 on] to S   82 in] one S
85 syknesses] S, syknesse C   it] Yet S   knowe] vnderstand princypally S
86 pryncipally] *om.* S   be] in S   87 suffocacyon] S, *om.* C   88 precipitation] + or
prefocacion C   matrice] + or dyslocacyon S   89 defaute] *om.* S   or] S, of C   90 is]
S, in C   cause] *om.* S   92 & ... her] S, *om.* C   93 joyned] S, joyneth C
97 deliueraunce] payne S   104 summe^2] + but S   while] well S

105 have hit surfetysly & anguisly & summe have hit lytyll wyle &
esly. And yf hit so be þat a woman have not hem euery monyth
onys fro þe tyme sche [may] [conceyve], þat ys fro xv yere till
sche be fyfty wyntyr olde, but yf hit be lettyd be eny of þeys
cavsys þat I shev here-aftyre, & but yf hit so be [that she be]
110 holpon be medycyn, sche schall passe suerly by on of þes iij
wayys. Othyr sche schall have a tesyk or sche schall fall in a
dropsy incurabyll or sche schall sodenly dey.

No'w' schell I tell yow wyche women may lese her flovrys
with-owtyn [dysesse] & þe cavse why they lese hem. Women þat
115 be with schyld have no flovrys be-cause þe schylde ys norschyde
in here body with [f. 5] þe same flovrys. [Ne tho that ben
grevously seke, for the seknes wasteth hir blode.] Ne tho þat
labure moche, for be þe sade labure of here body þey defey here
met þat þey receyve passyngely well. Ne tho þat syngvn & wake
120 mekyll, as do þes religios, for of her wakynge & travelynge in
syngynge here blode wastyth & defyet well here repast. Ne tho þat
have gret defavte of vytall, for here stomake & here lyuere been of
full poure for-to defey all þat þey receyve. Ne maydyns till þey be
xv yere olde, for þey be so yoyfull & so yonge þat here met
125 [defieth as] þei receyve hit, and þe blode [and] othyre humors so
byndynge & here vesell þat hit schulde passe by ys so smalle & so
strayte þat no thynge suche may passe. Ne þe women of l yerc [of]
age be-cause they be so dryed þat þe hote of þe blode is distroyde
þat no superhabundant humvre may ryse in hem ne passe.

130   Nov schall I tell yow why þys iij anguysch þat I spake of
by-fore [f. 5v] fallyn to women rathyre then to men. The fyrst
anguysch þat I spake of ys travelynge of chylde, & þat commyth

105 surfetysly] sore-fet B   107 may] BA, have D   conceyve] conceiue B,
conceyvy D   yere] + of age B   108 but yf] *om.* B   lettyd] + then B   eny] some B
109 that ... be] BA, *om.* D   110 medycyn] medicynes B   112 or] + ellys B
113 may] *om.* BA   114 dysesse] dyesse D, dissease B   115 be-cause] + that BA
116–17 Ne ... blode] B, *om.* D   117 Ne] Neiþer B   118 labure²] labourys B
120 religios] + folke B, women A   travelynge in] *om.* B   121 wastyth] + muche B
122 vytall] vitellis B   here²] *om.* B   125 defieth as] BA, þat D   and²] B, of D
126 so²] *om.* B   127 thynge suche] *tr.* BA   þe] these BA   of²] *om.* D   128 hote]
hete BA   129 superhabundant humvre] superhabundaunce of humours BA   ne passe]
om. B

105 syknesse fallith to a woman propirly at xv yeer of age, and fro that
tyme till fyfti yeer she may conceyue but it be lettyd be any of
thes causes her folwynge; and but she be holpen be medicynes,
she shal haue on of these thre: outhir she shal haue a tysyk, or a
dropsy oncurabill or ellis sodeynly dye.
110

The cause why women lese here flowres ar these. Women with
childe haue no floures for the child in here body is norished with
115 the same flowris, nor women that laboureth meche, for be sad
labour of here body they defye [þer] mete and drynke passyngely
well. Nor the women that weche, as do religious women, for of
here wakyng and labour in syngyng here blood wastith mekyll and
defieth here repaste. [f. 5] Nor tho women that wantyn vitaill, for
120 here stomakys and here lyuer are poore to defye that they
resseyue. Nor maydenys till they be xv yeer of age, for they are
joyefull and so yong her mete defyeth as they resseyue it. And so
the blood and other humoures passe a-way. Nor women of fyfty
yer of age, for they are so drye that hete of blood is wastyd that no
125 superhabundance of blood nor humoures may ryse in hem nor
passe.

130   Why these iij syknessis a-fore seyd falle to women rather than
to men. The firste is traueylyng of chyld, and that comyth of the
seed of man the which, receyuyd in here body, the child is

107 be medicynes] of the same causes S   108 thre] seknessis S   113 cause] causes S
114–15 for ... flowris] *om.* S   115 sad] *om.* S   116 þer] S, *om.* C   117 Nor] & S
the ... do] *om.* S   women²] + that wake mvche S   117–19 for ... repaste] *om.* S
121–22 for ... it] *om.* S   131 and] *om.* S   132 body] wherof S

of þe sede of man þe wyche woman receyuyth & in here body þe
chylde conceyuyth & so muste sche nedys have travill in
135 delyuerance, for þe wyche I can no medycyne writt. But sche þat
wol haue no travyll in chyldynge, let kepe here fro þe recevynge
of sede of man &, oon my parell, sche schall nevyre drede þe
travelynge of chylde.

The ij anguysch ys suffocacyon of matrice, þat is whan þe
140 matrice rysyth out of hys ry3ht plase & goyth ouer-hy, & þe cause
þer-of I schall schev yow by resonne. I have tolde yow here
be-fore þat þe matryce is made of synow & eche synov be kynde
ys colde & eche þinge þat ys colde sekyth hete, & þer-fore þe
matrice þat ys cold of hym-selfe, yf hit be not holp with oþer
145 thyngis, hit sekyth hete & so sume tymme hit goyth vp to þe most
hotest place of [f. 6] þe body of woman, þat ys þe hert, þe lyuyre,
þe mylte & þe longys, þe wyche cleue to-gedyre a-boute þe
stomack. And be-cause þat all þe breth þat we draw comyth by
contynuall clappynge of þe longis & whan þe matrice, þat ys full
150 of synovs, tochyth þe longis, hit pressyth hem & comburth hem
þat þey may not meve ne clappe for-to drav brethe & whan þe
breth may not in ne ovt, þe body ys as dede. & þat ys cause þat
women oþer-whyll ly a-svovnynge as þey were dede.

Precipitacion or prefocacion of matryce ys whan hit goyth out
155 of hys ry3ht place ouer-lov & þe cause of þat payne I schall tel
yow. There ys a bouell with-in þe body of manne & woman þat ys
clepid longaon, by þe wyche þe gret vryne passyth, of þe wyche
bouell þe on ende vpvarde ys yoynyde to þe stomak & þe oþer
ende donvarde ys yoynyde to þe ryge-bonys ende & at þe [f. 6v]
160 bladyr of man & woman, in þe wych vryne sympull ys gadderyde,
lyeth yoynyde to þe forseyde bovell dovnvarde; & summe-tyme
be diuerse causis þe synvys by þe wyche matryce ys fastenyde, for
ouer-mokyll moysture slakyn & vax longe & fallyn dovne & lyyth

---

133 woman] women B &] *om.* B 133–34 þe³ … conceyuyth] conceiveth þe
chylde B 134 travill] trauelyng B 137 of¹] + þe B 139 of] + the B 140 ouer-hy]
over the hert B 142 synow] synews B 148 be-cause] so causeth B 150 comburth]
encomberyth B, in combere A 152 not] + cvnme B ys²] + þe B 153 ly] + in B
154 Precipitacion or prefocacion] Prefocacioun or precipitacioun B hit] he B
156 of] + a B manne] + of a B 157 þe²] *twice* D 159 at] *om.* B

conceyuyd of, and ther-of muste she haue trauayle in
deliueraunce. Ffor this [ther] is no medycyne but kepe fro man.

135

The secunde syknesse is suffocacion of the matrice and that is
140   whan the matrice rysith [f. 5v] owte of the right place and goth
ouer-hye, and the cause is this. The matrice is made of thenne
skyn and senewis, the which of kynde are cold, and euery cold
thynge sekith hete, and therfore the matrice is cold of the self; if
'it' be not holpe with other thynges, it sekith hete and so sumtyme
145   it goth ouer-hye to the hottest place of the body, and that is the
herte, the lyver, the mylte and the lunges, the which cleue
to-gedire a-bowte the stomak. And be-cause the breth of a body
comyth be flappynge of the lungys, sumtyme the matrice in this
syknesse oppressith the lungys that thei may not meve and flappe
150   for-to drawe breth, and so whan the breth may nother in ne owte,
the body is as ded, and this is the cause that women ly othirwhile
[a-swone] as they wer ded.

Also prefocacion or precipitacion is whan the matrice risith
155   owte of the right place ouer-lowe and the cawse ther-of is a
certeyn bowel with-inne a man and woman callid longaon, be the
which the grete vryn passith, of the which bowel the ton ende
vpward is joyned to the stomak and the tother end dounward to the
reggebon end and the bladder of man and woman, in the which
160   vryn symple is gaderid, and therfore sumtyme be diuerse causis
the senewis that the matrice 'is' fastid by, be ouer-mykyl moyster
slakkyn and waxen longe and falle down and lye vpon þat bowel
and on the bladder and will not suffre the vryn symple to come

133 of¹] *om.* S   134 ther] S, *om.* C   kepe] + her S   139 that] it S   141 of] + a S
143 is] beenge S   the²] it S   144 hete] helpe S   152 a-swone] eswone C, in
swoune S   156 and] or S   159 in] to S   160 symple] symply S   162 slakkyn]
slakked S   163 the²] + gret S   symple] *om.* S

vp-on þat bouell & on þe bladyre, þe wyche may not devly þe
165   vrynne sympull receyue, hold, ne lette passe, & op-pressyth so þe
gret bouell þat þe gret vrine may haue no resonabull yssev. And so
be þe causis grete dysessys fallvn to þe bladdere & bouellys & to
þe reynes & þe gret vrynne þat may noon yssev have [casteth] vp
a gret fume to þe hede & trovbelyth þe braynne & makyth þe hed
170   to ake & þe pacient to lese all talent of mete & drynke & of
naturall reste, to slepe.

        The iij anguysch ys retencyon, defaute or superfluite of flouris.
But fyrst I woll tell yow where-of the [f. 7] flouris comme & þan
schall I tell yow þe cause of retencyon & defaut & þe cause of
175   superfluyte of hem & þan schall I tell [you] þe medycyn for eche
of hem. The cause of here commynge ys þys: alle þe mete þat we
receyue goyth in-to þe stomak and þer hit ys sodune & defyede &
all þat ys gret & not profitabull to man passyth dovne be þe
[bowell] þat ys clepit longaon & þer passyth hit a-vay & þat þat ys
180   pure & clene a-bydyth in þe stomak & þer hit ys turnyde in-to þe
substans of mylk & þat substans passyth to þe lyuere & þer hit is
a-noþer tyme defyede & sodyn & full well clensyde, and all þat is
not profitabull descendit vn-to þe bladdere & ys callyde vrynne
sympull. But þe remenavnt þat ys good [and] clere abydyth on þe
185   lyuere & þer tornyth in-to blode & so fro þens hit passyth to all
membyrs of a mannys body & so norschyth hys lyffe.

        And sethen þe [f. 7v] lyuere & þe stomak of þe most hottest
man been besy j-now to sethe & defy þe mete þat he receyuyth &
þe drynke, and þe moste coldeste man ys more hottere þan þe
190   most hotest woman, how schulde þan þey defy here mete clene þat
þey receyve? Hit myȝth not be donne be way of reson but at euery
repaste of necessyte þer abydyth summe thyng on þe liuere
undefyed & tho superfluiteys dravn hem to-gedyre in-to a vessell
þat ys ordende for hem, þat hath hys one ende joynyde to þe lyuer

164 þat] þe B   166 no] noon B   resonabull] conuenient B, comendabell A
168 casteth] B, cast A, castynge D   169 fume] swyme B   &¹] *om.* BA   170 of²]
all B   173 þan] *om.* B   174 schall I] *tr.* B   175 you] B, *om.* D   179 bowell] BA,
bouellys D   180 turnyde] turneth BA   181 þat] the B   182 þat] *twice* D   183 &]
+ it B   184 and] BA, *om.* D   188 &¹] + to B   189 man] + þat is B   190 þan þey]
tr. BA   191 be²] + no BA   193 undefyed] not defied B   194 þat²] + hauen B   one]
over BA

and passe, and so it oppressith the bowel that the gret vryn may
165   haue non yssew, wherof fallith gret dissese [f. 6v] to the bowell, to
the bladdere and to þe reynes. And the gret vryn that may non
jssew haue castith vp a gret fume onto the hed and troublith the
brayn and makith þe hed to ake and the pacient to lese talent of
mete and drynke and naturall reste.
170

The thirde syknesse is retencion, defawte [or] superfluite of
flowris, but firste vnderstonde wherof the floures come and
aftirward retencion, defawte and cavse of here superfluite. The
175   cause of comyng of floures is this: all the mete and drynke that is
receyuyd goth in-to þe stomak and ther it is sodyn and defyed.
And all that is gret and not profitabill passith down be the bowell
callid longaon, and `þer´ bidith in the stomak and ther tornyth in-to
mylke and so passith into the lyuer and ther a-bidith till it be
180   defyed and sodyn and wel clensyd. And all that is not
profita[f. 7]bill, passith to the reynes, into the bladder and so owte.
And that is callid vryn symple; but that is good a-bidyth in þe
lyuer and ther turnyth to blood and so fro thens it passith to all the
humours of the body, and noryshith the lyf.
185

And syn the stomak and the liuer of þe hottest man ar besy
jnowh to sethe & defye mete and drynke that he resseyuyth, how
shulde women defye here foode syn the coldest man is hottere
than the hottest woman, the which they may not do be reson, but
190   at euery repaste of necessite a-bideth sum thyng on ther liuer
vndefyed, the which growith to superfluites and drawe to-gedir
in-to a vessel ordend for hem, of whech on ende is joyned to the
lyuer and the nedir ende to the navill of þe woman, joyned to here

165 bowell] + & S   167 haue] hathe & S   fume] fome S   172 or] of C   defaute ...
superfluitc] *om.* S   174 defawte ... superfluite] therof S   177 be] to S   178 þer] that
yt   and ther] *om.* S   179 it] he S   180 and¹] *om.* S   181 reynes] + & S   187 syn]
seeng S   the²] *om.* S   189 syn] seeng S

195 & hys oþer to þe navyll of þe woman, joynyde to þe matrice, so
þat þe superfluytes rottvn in þat vessell & tvrnyth in-to a mortall
venym. But nature, þat hatyth euery corrupcion & voydyth afthyre
hys povere all þynge þat is [noyant] to body of man, enforsyth
euery monyth onys to purge & clense þe body of euyll humorys &
200 corrupte. And so þis purgacyon ys ordende to women & ys clepid
[f. 8] menstrual be-cause hit commyth euery monyth onys. And þe
more hottere þe woman ys of compleccyon, þe lasse schall sche
have of here flourys.
         Now schall I tell yow þe cause of retencyon & fa'y'llynge of
205 floures. Hit fallit oþer-whyle of defaute of blode & þat commyth
to a woman þat ys hote & dry of complexion, in wyche þe blode
ys mochyll vastyde, & þat ys þe cause þat þey be lene & make
mochyll urine & so þe flourys be holdvnne. And oþer-whyll hit
commyth of þat þe blode ys stopyde, þat hit may haue no yssev, &
210 þat commyth of colde & of drynesse. For bothe qualites mak þe
vaynes narov, small & strayte. And oþer-whyle hit commyth of
gret congeylynge of blode þat for þe grosnesse hit may not passe
þe vaynes, & þat befallyth whan melancholy ys cause of þat
defaut; & ye schall knov þe dysesse whan [a] woman makyth but
215 lytyll watyre & thyn. And oþer-whyle hit fallyth by-cause þat þe
blode þat scholde go þere a-way [f. 8v] passyth by o-þer wayys, as
be vomyt or bledynge at þe nose or þe emeroydys be-nethe, & þat
ys of þe flovyre þat sekyth to have yssev & may haue nonne & so
voydyth there. And yf hit stope be-cause hit may have no
220 resonabull yssev, ye schall mak hem hole be medycyns þat sewyn
here-aftyre, where hit spekyth yf women have to lytyll of here
flourys.
         Now schall I tell yow þe causys þat makyn þe flowrys to fall to
superhabundantly & ovte of co'v'rs. j cause ys þat þe vaynes of þe

194–95 joynyde … woman] *om.* B   198 noyant] B, noyand A, noryschant D
199 humorys] humour B   199–200 & corrupte] *om.* B   200 to] for B   202 þe¹]
that a B   204 yow] *om.* B   205 of¹] for BA   &] *om.* B   206 of] in B   207 þe]
by B   þat²] *om.* BA   210 bothe] + þoo B, + þes A   212 grosnesse] grettnesse BA
214 þe] þat BA   a] BA, *om.* D   215 hit fallyth] *om.* B   217 vomyt] woundis B
218 flovyre] flowrys B   220 sewyn] shewen B   221 yf] of B   have] hauyng B
224 j] *om.* B

195 matrice, so that the superfluites rotyn in that vessell and turne
in-to corrupcion. But than nature, that hatith euery [f. 7v]
corrupcion, voidith at his power all thyn'g' that noyeth the body of
man or woman, and enforsith euery monyth onys to purge and
clense the body of ille humoures and corrupcion. So this
200 purgacion fallith to woman and is callid menstrualis be-cause it
comyth euery monyth onys. And the hotter that woman is, the
lesse she shal haue of hir floures.

    The cause of retencion and faylynge of the floures ffallith
205 othir-while for defawte of blood and þat comyth to a woman that
is hot and drye of complexion, in which blood is meche wastyd,
and that is [the] cawse thei are lene and mak mekill vryn and so
here floures are with-hold. And sumtyme it fallith that the blood is
stoppyd, that it may non jssew haue, and that comyth of cold and
210 drynesse, for tho too qualites make the veynes narwe, smale and
streyte. And othir-while it fallith of congelynge of blood [f. 8] that
for thyknesse it may not passe þe veynes, and that makith
malencoly; that dishese ye may knowe for the woman makith litill
water and thenne. And sumtyme it fallith of blood that shuld ther
215 a-way passith be other weyes, as be vometis, be bledynge at the
nose or be þe emerawdys be-nethe, and that is of the floures that
sekith jssew and may non haue but there, and yif thei stoppe
be-cause they may haue no resnabill issu, ye may hele hem with
medycines rehersid her-after.
220

    The causes that makith the flours to falle oute of course. On
cause is that the veynes of the matrice are ofte tyme ouer-open,

---

196 than] that S   197 at] with S   199 corrupcion] + & S   204 the] *om.* S
205 blood] bloudis S   and] when S   207 the] S, *om.* C   209 may] + have S   haue]
om. S   210 narwe] + & S   214 and] *om.* S   215 ther a-way] pas that way & S   be']
om. S   217 haue] + 'it' S   224 cause] *om.* S   tyme] *om.* S

225   matryce been oftvn tyme ouer-opyn & þat schall be know whan þe
       flovyre passyth hastyly rede & clere. An-oþir cause ys whan a
       woman hath gaderyde ouer-moche blode by ouer-moche mete &
       ouer-moche drynck & ouer-moche reste and oþer-whyll hit
       commyth be-cause [the] blode ys ouyre-moche chavfyde be colere
230   or oþer humors þat cvme oute of þe hede & oþer partyes of þe
       body & medyll with [f. 9] þe blode & chaufe hit & mak hit to
       boyle [þat] þe vaynes may not hold hit. And yf þe flovrys þat
       passvn comme of colere, þan þey be yelov. And yf þey comme of
       blode, þan be þey rede & yf þey comme of flevme, þan be þey
235   watyre-lycke & pale.

          An-oþer cause þer ys be-cause þat all þat blode with-in þe body
       of woman ys corrupte thynge & nature of hys pouere woll woyde
       corrupte thyngys [and noyant] to mannys body & womannys
       & so makyth þe flovrys to [voyde to] superhabundantly &
240   ouyre-owtragisly, so þat hit makyth þe [woman] to lese talent to
       mete & drynck, & makyth here so febull þat here lyuere coldyth
       for þe blode þat sche lesyth & may not a-byde in hys kendly
       'h'ete, ne to defy þe mete & drynck in-to kyndly blode, but turnyth
       so in-to vatyre & fallyth to a dropsy in-curabyll, but yf þey be þe
245   sonnere j-holpyn & stopyde by medycynys þat ye schall fynde
       here-aftere where [f. 9v] hit spekith for superfluite of ouer-moche
       flovrys. I have tolde yow here-before why the women fayle
       flowrys or ellys have ry3th feve, & þe cause.

          Now schal I tell yow at what age a mayden may vse resonably
250   þe dedyut of dewery. Euery mayde schulde kepe here fro þe
       dedyut at þe leste telle here flovrys be fall & comyn, þat ys till
       sche be xv yere olde, þat nature & þe ma't'rys myth fulfyll & bere
       þat þat longith to hem of kynde, for trewly & sche vse dedyut or
       þat tyme, on of þeys iij thyngis or all schall fall to here. Othyre

---

225 be] ye B   226 flovyre] flourys B   clere] + And B   227 ouer-moche¹] grett &
over mykyll B   227–28 & ouer-moche] *om.* B   229 the] B, of D   chavfyde]
chaunged B   231 chaufe] chaseth B   232 þat¹] that B, with D   234 be þey] *tr.* BA
236 cause] *om.* B   238 noyant] B, noyschant D, noyssant A   239 voyde to] B, *om.* D
240 woman] B, women D   244 to] into BA   þey] she BA   246 for] + þe BA   of
ouer-moche] or moche of B   247 yow] *om.* B   why the] whiche B   249–50 vse …
dewery] resonable vse to dele with man B   251 dedyut] man B   253 of kynde] *om.* B
dedyut] to dele with man B

225 and that ye may knowe whan the floures passe ouer-hastily red
and cleer. Another cawse is whan woman gadrith ouer-meche
blood be meche mete and drynk and ouer-mech reste. And
sumtyme it comyth be-cause the blood is [ouer-]moche chafyd be
coleryk or other humours that [f. 8v] if it come owte of the hed
230 and other partis of the body and medyll with the blood and chafe it
so to boyle that the veynes may not hold it. And yif the flour that
passe come of coleryk, than they are yelew. And yif they come of
the blood, þei are red. And yif thei come of flewme, thei are watir-
lyke and pale.
235

An-other cawse ther is, whan blood with-in the body is
corrupte, than nature at his power voydith corrupte thynges and
noyand to the body of man and woman, and so makith floures to
passe [superhabundantly], so that it makith a woman to lese talent
240 of mete and drynke, and febillith here so sore that hire lyver
coldith for the blood þat she lesith, which may not a-byde in his
keendely hete to defye mete and drynke into kendly blood, but
turnyth so in-to watir and fallith to a dropsy vncurabill, but she be
the sunner holpe and stoppid be medycines for superfluyte and
245 ouer-mekill of floures.

[f. 9] At what age a woman may vse hire body naturaly with
250 man. Clerkis sey at xv yeer of age and not a-fore, to saue
here-silff. Ffor euery mayde shulde kepe hire-self fro that deede
till here flouris be falle, and that is comonly at xv yeer of age, and
than aftir that nature and the matrice myght holde that longith to
hem of keende. Ffor truly yif she vse that deede with man a-for

226 woman] women S   228 ouer] S, oue C   229 if] + that C   230 chafe] cane not
sethe S   232 of²] to S   yif] *om.* S   they²] + that S   233 the] *om.* S   238 noyand]
noysom S   239 superhabundantly] S, superhabuntanly C   241 for] + lake of the S
243 turnyth] turns it S   244 supcrfluytc] superfluites S   250 yeer] yers S
253 myght] may S

255 sche schall be baren, or ellys here brethe schall have evyll sauor,
     or sche schall be to lauy of here body to oþer þan to here
     hosbande. But for þe fyrst I schall fynde medecyn here-aftere; þe
     iij ys in-curabylle.
         Now schall I tell yow whyche women be most abyll to
260 conceyue and [f. 10] whan: tho þat be purgyde of clene blode &
     not to mokyll. And tho þat have þe movth of here matrice nygh
     and euyn a-gayn þe wyket of here wombe. And tho þat haue þe
     body not ouyre-hard ne ouer-softe & been of good colovre &
     iocvnde & mery, and go not to þat play whan here wombe ys
265 ouer-replet. And a lytill be-fore or a sone afture here flourys is
     most conuenyant tyme & best to conceyve.
         Now schall I tell yow how whomen schall kepe hem whan þey
     knov þey have conceyuyde. Loke þey kepe them restely & wol not
     ouer-gretly trauell here body, ne wit rydynge nothyre with
270 ouer-moche goynge, ne þat þey be not sterid to ouer-moche
     angyre ne wrath & in þe vij monyth let kepe here esyly, for þan ys
     þe chylde formyde & be ouyr-mokyll sterynge of þe woman hit
     myȝth lytely passe or be myˈsˈschapyn, for [f. 10v] as I schall scew
     yow here-afture by reson, a chyld may be borvnne in þe vij
275 monyth, & þer-for hit ys nedfull for þe woman to kepe well þe
     partyes be-nethe for handelynge or chavfynge of hem by
     ouyre-mochyll goyng or rydynge or ony oþer thyng; & namly þat
     sche gyrde here not to strayte vndyre here brystys but hold here
     þer as slack as sche can & þat here brystys be at large to fill þem
280 full of mylk, for many desesys may fall to a woman for ouer-strait
     byndyng in þe vij monyth. But principali loke þey kepe hem well
     in þe viij monyth, for þan be þey heuy & grett; lett hem than kepe
     hem & reste & ete mesurably & kepe here wombe at large &
     anoynt hit with oyle [ceprine] or with oyle olyff or with oyle

255 have] + an B   256 to¹] *om.* B   257 I … fynde] ther been B   medecyn
here-aftere] medicynes and for the secund but B   258 in-curabylle] vncurable BA
261–62 nygh and] right B   263 &²] *om.* B   265 ouer-replet] replete B   a¹] *om.* B
266 conuenyant] conuenable B, commendabyl A   268 wol] vse B   269 ouer-gretly]
over grett B   trauell] + with B   ne] nether B   nothyre] ne B   270 ouer-moche¹]
much B   271 angyre] wrathe B   wrath] angwyshe B   272 hit] the chylde B
282 be þey] *tr.* B   than] *om.* B   283 hem] + than B   &¹] in B   284 with …
ceprine] *om.* B   ceprine] ceroine D

255 that age, on of these thre thynges shal falle to here: outher she shal
be bareyn, or ellis here breth shal stynke and haue an ylle savour,
or ellis she shal be lavy of here body. But for the ij ferste ye may
haue medicynes heer-aftir.

Knowe heer what women ar moste abill to conceyue and
260 whanne: tho women that are purgid of here corrupte blood and not
to meche, and tho that haue the mowth of þe matrice nygh and
even a-yens þe privite [f. 9v] of the wombe. And tho that haue
ther body not ouer-hard nor ouer-softe and are of good colour,
jocond and mery, and go not [to] that pley whan here wombe is
265 replete. Also a litill a-fore or sone aftir that hire floures are past is
beste tyme to conceyue.

How women shal kepe hem whan they knowe hem conceyuyd
with chyld. Loke that they kepe hem restly and vse not here body
with ouer-meche labour, or rydynge or goynge, nor that they be
270 not steryd to ouer-meche anger and wrath. And in the vij monyth
lete here [labour] esyly, for than is the childe fourmed, and be
ouer-meche sterynge of the wombe it myght lyghtly passe or ellis
be mysshapyn, for as ye shal vnderstond here-after, a child may be
born in the vij monyth. And therfore a woman owhte to kepe here
275 wel in the parties be-nethe fro handelyng or chafynge of hem be
mech rydynge or goynge, and othir gret labours. [f. 10] And
namely thanne that she girdith here not to streyte vndir the brestis,
but slak so that hire brestis may be at large to felle hem of mylke.
Ffor many dishesis may falle to a woman of ouer-streyte gyrdynge
280 in the vij monyth, but principally thei kepe hem wel in the viij
monyth, for than thei are heuy and grete; than lete hem kepe hem
in reste and ete mesurably and kepe here wombe at large and
a-noynte it with oyle [cypryne] or oyle olyf or oyle [mirtyn] and
kepe hem wel whan the child sterith. And in the ix monyth lete

256 ylle] evell S   262 tho] they S   264 go] *om.* S   to] *om.* CS   265 a-fore]
before S   268 restly] esily S   271 labour] S, *om.* C   280 thei] lett them S
282 kepe] lett S   wombe] + þe S   283 cypryne] cyroyne CS   mirtyn] nortyn C,
norteyne S

285 [mirton] & kepe hem well whan þe chylde steryth. And in þe ix
monyth lok þey kepe hem slak beneth & bynde hem [f. 11] hard
vndyre here pappys with a brode gyrdill; þan whan þe chyld
dravth donward he reyseth [not] vp a-gayne [ne] torne hym
a-mysse. & vse plastrys & bathys & oynementys of þe sewet of a
290 dere or of a gott be-nethe at here weket, þe movth of þe matrice to
enlarge, & þat in þat tyme sche entermet hyre not with no disport
of [deduyt] & namly ny here tyme, for with suche puttynge þe
secundynne myght brek & so þe chylde be abortyffe and stroyde
for euyre.
295   And yf ye woll know what ys a secvndyne, I schall tell yow.
Ry`g´th as ye se in a egge þe chekyn ys wrappyde in a lythill thyn
skynne, ry3th so þe chylde lyeth wrappyde in þe modyre wombe
in such a lityll skynne, þe whyche he brekith & bryngyth forth
with hym whan he ys borvnne. And yf hytt a-bydyth with-in & be
300 not browth forthe be medycynys, þat ye schall [f. 11v] se in þys
bok where he tretyth of þe delyverance of þe secundine.
         An abortyffe ys a chylde þat ys dede in hys modere wombe.
The sygnes of þe wyche ye schall know be theys. The brestys of
þe woman wol wex small & lene and oft sche felyth dysesse as
305 sche scholde travell of chylde be-fore comenabill tyme, & sche
felythe gret cold in here reynys, & a black vrine passyth
oþer-whyle at here wyket & at þe last þer a-peryth a black skyn or
elys a dede chylde, & þat may fall be smytynge or be fallynge.
And summe women vsyn a þynge for they schold not conceyve &
310 þat makyth abortyf, & slen hem-selfe al-so, the whych I dare not
wryte lest sume cursyde calet wold hit vse.
         Now woll I tell yow what may lette a woman with chylde of
ry3ht dclyuerance. Sche may be dystrovbelyd yf sche be angury or

---

285 mirton] B, *lacuna in* D   287 þan] that B   288 reyseth] resorte BA   not] BA,
om. D   ne] B, ner A, *om.* D   289 sewet] swet B   290 here weket] the entre of hir
wombe B   290–91 þe … enlarge] to enlarge the mowthe of her matrice B   þat¹]
om. B   tyme] + that   292 of] or B   deduyt] deuyt D, delyng with man B, drwry A
293 secundynne] + or skynne B   295 a] the BA   296 wrappyde] warpid B
301 secundine] + the chylde shall be abortyfe B, What is abortyf and what be his
signes A   302 An] And B   303 ye … know] *om.* B   306 a] *om.* B   307 wyket]
wombe B   308 be²] *om.* B   310 slen] to slee B   al-so] + þer been medicynes B
313 be dystrovbelyd] distroye hit B

285   hem kepe hem slak be-nethe, and bynde hem harde [vnder the]
       pappis with a brood girdill, that whan the child drawith
       downward, he ryse not vpward a-yen and turne hym mys. And vse
       bathis, plaistris and onymentis of suet of a deer or of a got
       be-nethe at hire priuyte to enlarge the mowth of the matrice, and
290   that she dispose [f. 10v] not here body naturally with man, namely
       ny here tyme, ffor with that werke she myght breke the secundyne
       and so the child myght be abortiff and distroyed.

295   What is the secundyne, ye may knowe. Lyke as ye se in an eg
       the cheken wrappid in a thenne skyn, right so the child ly[t]h
       wrapped in the modris wombe in a litill skin, the which he brekith
       and bryngith foorth with hym at his berth. And if it a-byde and be
       not brought forth be medycines that ye shal fynde in this book, she
300   shal stonde in gret perell of deth.

    What is abortiff. Abortif is a childe ded in the moodris wombe.
       The signes wherof ye shal knowe: the brestes of the woman will
       wax smale and leene, and often she felith dishese as she shuld
305   trauayle of child afore comenabill tyme, and she felith gret cold in
       here reynes, and she makith other-whyle blak vryn, and at the
       laste [f. 11] ther aperith a blak skyn or ellis the child ded, and that
       may falle of smytynge or be fallynge, or mysgydynge of her-self.

310

    Dyuers thynges may lette a woman to haue good deliueraunce.
       On is, yif she be angry, prowde, shame-faste, or ellis if it be here

---

285 hem[1]] + hard vnder the pappis *crossed through* C   harde] fast S   vnder the] S,
vnde C   287 mys] amysse S   296 ly[t]h] lyh C, lyethe S   299 forth] owt S
302 Abortif] It S   305 comenabill] convenient S   308 be] *om.* S   of[2]] *om.* S
313 prowde] + or S

prowde or scham[f. 12]full, or ellys þat hit be here fyrst chylde, or
315 ellys þat sche be small & megyr of body or ellys ouer-fatt, or þat
þe matryce be febyll or in ouyre-gret het or elys þat chylde be
dysturbyde with summe knot in þe nek of þe matrice or els þat þe
movthe of þe marys be to clos or tornyde in þe on syde or on þe
othyre, or ellys yf sche have þe stonne, or ellys yf here bovell be
320 ouer-replet of þe gret vrynne for defaute of dygestyon, or ellys yf
þe chylde have ouer-gret a hede or body, or [if he haue oþer
membres then he sholde haue of reasoun, or] yf hit hathe dropsy
or oþer euyls, or dede, or turnyde a-gayn kynde.

   Now have I tolde yow þe lettynge of redy & tymfull
325 delyuerance of chylde. Now woll I wˈrˈyth to yow medycynys for
redy delyuerance yf hit be here tyme. Whan a woman travelyth &
here throwys commyth, take þe rotys of polypodye þat growth on
þe oke & stampe hym & bynde hem vndyre þe solys of here fete,
& the [f. 12v] chyld schall be borne all-thow he be dede. Or tak þe
330 sede of wilde commyn as hit grovyth in þe herbe, & afture tak
woll þat [grovyth] in þe myddys of þe frownt of a chepe, & medill
þe sede & þat to-gedyr & whan nede ys bynde hit to hare raynes.
But as sone as sche ys delyuerde, take hit away or ellys þe matrice
will sew aftyr hit. An-othyre: tak lek bladys & scalde hem & as
335 hote as sche may suffyre hem, bynde hem to here navyll & þey
woll delyuere here a-nonne all-thowhe þe chyld be dede; but tak
hem a-way afture þe delyuerance a-noon or ellys all hare bovellys
will sew aftyre.

   How ye schall help a woman þat [trauelyth] of chylde. Fyrst ye
340 schall vndyrstonde þat [in iij] maners chyldervn mow schew hem
resonabyly at here byrth. For oþer þey schew hare hede and hare
fete, or þe oon syde, or þe oþer, or þe hede & þe fete yontly to

314 ellys þat] if B, if it A   315 &] or B   or ellys] other B   or²] other B
317 dysturbyde] desturbylyd A , distrobled B   318 marys] matrice B   in] over B,
on A   319 ellys²] *om.* BA   320 þe] so B   321 a] hand B   321–22 if … or] B, or yf
þey have more membris þan it shold haue be resson A, *om.* D   323 turnyde] turne B
325 to] *om.* B   for] of B   329 be borne] come B   330 in] on B   331 grovyth]
grovth D, groweth B   332 whan … ys] if nede be   336–37 all-thowhe … a-noon]
om. B   337 hare] þe B   338 sew] shewe B folow A   339 schall] sholde B
trauelyth] B, travelyd D   340 in iij] iiij D, iij BA   hem] + selfe B   341 and] or B
342 þe³] ther B   þe⁴] her B   yontly] ioyned B

firste child, or yif she be smal and megre of body or ouer-fat, or if
315 the matrice be febill or in ouer-gret hete. Or ellis if the child be
disturbyd with any knot in the nekke of the matrice, or yif the
mowthe of the matrice be to close, or be turned on the ton syde, or
on the tothir, or yif she haue the ston, or yif here bowel be
ouer-replete of the gret vryn for defawte of digestion, or yif the
320 child haue ouer-gret an hed or a body, or yif he haue mo membris
than he shuld haue of reson, or if it haue the dropsy or othir euyll,
or ded, or turned a-yen kende.

These are the lettyngis at redy tyme of childyng. [f. 11v]
325 Medicines to make redy diliueraunce of child at tyme whan a
woman trauailith and here throwys come. Take the rootis of
polipodye and stampe hem and bynde hem vnder the solys of here
feet, and the child shal be born thowgh it be ded. Or ellis tak the
seed of wylde comyn as it groweth on the erbe, and than take
330 wulle that growith a-myddis in the fronte of a sheep; do thes ij
to-gedir, and whan neede is bynde it to here reynes, but as sone as
she is deliuerid, take it a-wey or ellis the matrice will sue aftir it.
Also a-nother: take leek bladis and skalde hem and as hot as she
may suffre, bynde hem to here navyll and thei will deliuer here
335 a-non thowgh the child be ded; but tak hem a-way a-non after
deliueraunce, for ell all [her bowellis] will come after.

How ye shal helpe the woman whan she trauaylith. Ffirste ye
340 shal vnderstande that in iij maners [f. 12] a child may shewe hym
resonably at his birth. Ferste otherwhile he shewith his hed,
sumtyme his feet, sumtyme the ton syde, sumtyme the tother, and

316 any] one S   317 on] vnto S   319 ouer-replete] full S   320 he] it S   321 he] it S
330 a-] in þe S   in] of S   334 thei ... here] she shalbe delyuerid S   336 her bowellis]
S, *om.* C   come] + owt S

gydyre. [f. 13] But oþer casys mow othyre-whyle fall for tho þat
schew fyrst here hede, þey have peraventure all þe remmenavnt of
345   here body to þe oon syde or to þat oþer, þat whan þe hede ys in þe
nek of þe matrice, hys nek lyeth ouerthwart with-in & oþer-whyle
he puttyth forth hys on honde & the remnavnt a-bydyth with-yn.
And svmme-tyme hys oon fote & summe-tyme hys both & hys
hondys joyntly to-gethyre, and svme-tyme he fastenyth hys oo
350   fote or ellys bothe hys fete to þe sydys of þe wyket be-for or
be-hynde & þat oo syde or þe othyre. And oþer-whyle he hath hys
hondys a-bove on hys hede, and sume-tyme he puttyth hys fete to
þe syde of þe matryce & þer ys he fastenyde. And svme-tyme he
schevyth hys kneys & svm-tyme hys bottokkys.
355   And svm-tyme hit ys so þat ye schall fynde hys fete joynyd in
þe neck of þe matryce. And be-cause þat many [f. 13v] women
perysch for defavte of connynge helpe & good, y schall tell yow
how ye schall helpe hem at nede.
         But furste y schall wryth [moo] medycyns for delyuerance of
360   chyde. Yeue hare to drynk þe schavynge of yuery & sche schall
chylde & do þe same to on þat spekyth in hys sleppe. For-to mak a
woman sonne to be delyverd of chyde, [whethyre] hit be quyk or
dede, ȝeff hare to drynk dytayn, to drammys, with þe watyre of
fenygrek & ȝef here to ete dyamergariton & sche schall be
365   delyuerde. For þe same a-noþer medyson preuyde ofte tymys
trew: tak of myrre, þe quantite of j hasull not, & ȝyf here to drynk
in wynne & with-owtyn fayl sche schall be delyuerd a-noon. And
yf þe chylde be dede, ȝef here to drynk ysop & hote watere & sone
schall sche be delyuerde. Or tak a lytyll scrowe & wryt þys
370   with-in: + In nomine Patris et Filij & Spiritus Sancti Amen +
Sancta Maria + Sancta [f. 14] Margareta + ogor + sugor + nogo +

343 casys] causes B, caus A   othyre-whyle] other B   347 hys] *om.* B   348 hys²]
om. BA   350 ellys] *om.* B   hys] *om.* B   sydys] syde B   wyket] mouthe of þe
wombe B   351 & þat] on the B   352 on] *om.* B   fete] fote B   353 &] *om.* B
354 bottokkys] buttok B   357 perysch] + children B   359 moo] BA, my D
360 chyde] D, chylde B   362 whethyre] whehyre D, wheþer B   364 ete] drynk B
366 trew] *om.* B   of¹] *om.* B   j] an B, a A   367 in] with B   368 &¹] in B
369 schall sche] *tr.* B   scrowe] strowe B   371 sugor] *om.* B

sumtyme his hed and his feet joyntly to-gedir. But other [cases]
may othirwhile falle to that. Whan he shewith firste his hed,
345 peraventour he hath alle þe remanentis of his body to the ton syde
or to the tother, so that whan his hed is in the nekke of the matrice,
his necke lyth ouer-thwert with-inne, and sum-tyme he puttith
owte his on hande and [the] remanent a-bidith with-inne. And
sumtyme he puttith his on foot and sumtyme bothe, and sumtyme
350 he hath hys handis a-boue his hed, and sumtyme he puttith his feet
to the sydes of the matrice and ther is he [fastenyd], and sumtyme
he shewith his knees and sumtyme his buttok.

355 And sumtyme ye shal fynde his feet joyned in the necke of the
matrice, and therof many [f. 12v] women perish for fawte of
cunnynge and good helpe. To helpe all these ye shal knowe heer
aftirward.
But firste ye shal see mo medicynes for diliueraunce of child.
360 Whan she shal trauayle, gyf here [to] drynke the chafyng of yvery,
and she shal childe. And do that same to any that spekith in here
sleep. Also to redy deliueraunce, whedir the child be quyk or ded,
yeue here drynke dytayne ij ʒ with water of ffenygrek and yeue
here diamargariton and she shal be deliuerid. Also for hasty
365 deliueraunce, whether the child be quyk or ded, for it hath ofte be
provyd. Take myrre, the quantite of a note, and yeue it here to
drynke in wyne and she shal sone be deliuerid. And yif the child
be ded in the modris wombe, yeue here drynke jsop in hot watir
and she shal sone be deliuerid. And write in a skrowe all the
370 psalme of Magnificat [f. 13] and gerde hit a-bowte here. But wit
wel that this nor non othir helpith a woman at comenabill tyme of

343 joyntly] joyned S   cases] S, cas C   344 othirwhile falle] *tr.* S   that] as S
348 the] S, *om.* C   351 the¹] oon S   is he] *tr.* S   fastenyd] S, fastid C   356 many]
may S   fawte] lake S   360 to] S, *om.* C   361 that¹] the S   362 to] for S   363 of]
om. S   364-6 Also ... provyd] or ellis S   366 quantite] greatnes S   368 the] hes S
369 skrowe] scrowle S   370-72 wit ... with] yet ye medwiff most doe S

and kyt þat scrov in-to small pecys & ȝiffe here to drynk. Or wrytt
in a longe scrow all þe psalme of Magnificat anima mea & gyrde
hit a-boute here. But wethyth well þat þis ne nonne oþer kepyth no
375   woman   at   commenabyll   tyme   of   delyuerance   [but   as   a
preparatyue] & þer-for let þe mydwyffe helpe.

ȝif hit so be þe chylde fyrste schevyth hys hede & þe remenavnt
of hys body cleue to þe oon syde, þan put to yowur honde &
dresse hym þat bothe hys hondys ley yontly to hys sydes, so þat
380   he may comme ryth forth. And whan he schewyth bothe hys
leggys joyntly, put to yowur hond and sese hym be þe fote & draw
hym forth a-vysydly, þat he be not dysiontyde, & þat he opyn not
hys handys & cleue vn-to þe sydys of þe nek of þe matryce.

385   And yf hit be so that hys hede be so gret þat hit may not ovte,
put to yowur honde & [f. 14v] put hym a-gayne in & a-noynte þe
movthe [of the] matryce with softe oynementis, as ys oyle oleve or
oyle de bay. And let þe myddewyffe whete hare [handys] in
watyre þat fenygrek & lynnesede haue be sodon in; þan sese þe
390   hede & draw hym so forth.

And yf þe chylde ley a-gaynne kynde, lette þe modere ley on a
herde bede, so þat sche have here hede & hare scholdrys wel hy,
& þan a-vysydly & well put to yowur honde & dresse hym so þat
he comme forthe in dew maner & so draw hym forth; but loke in
395   þe mene whyle sche ley oon a herde bedde.

And yf he holde with þat oon hand, lok ye draw hym not forth,
than ye myȝght dysioynte hym, but set yowur fyngere on hys
scholdrys & so put hym yn a-gayne & dresse hys handys to hys
syde & þan tak hym by þe hede & draw hym softe forth. And yf
400   he hold bothe hys handys, put yowur oon hande on þat oon

---

372 scrov] strowe B   373 scrow] strowe B   mea] + dominum B   374 wethyth] ye
shall knowe B   no] medicyne helpyth any B   375 commenabyll] conuenable B
375–76 but ... preparatyue] B, *om.* D   377 be] + that   378 honde] handis B
381 fote] feete B   382 a-vysydly] wisely BA   þat he] *om.* B   383 &] for fere þat
they B   385 so²] to B   386 agayne in] *tr.* B   387 of the] BA, *om.* D   388 handys]
handis B, handes A handym D   391 ley¹] be B   392 scholdrys] + lieng B, lyth A
393 þan] + wel B   a-vysydly] avisely B   394 he] + may BA   394–95 & ... bedde]
om. B   396 þat] the B   forth] for B   397 set] putte B   fyngere] fyngers B
400 þat] the B

deliueraunce and therfore let euery mydwyf helpe with her besynesse.

375

Now of the birthe of a childe. Yif so be the childe shewe first his hed and the remanent of the body cleue to the syde, than puttith to youre hand and dresse hym that both his handis ly
380 joyntly to his sydes, so that he may come right foorth. And yif he shewe bothe his leggis ioyntly, than put to your hand and sese hym be the feet and drawe hym forth wysely, that he be not [dysioynted] in his armys, and þat he open not his handis and cleue to the matrice, but dresse wysely to his sydes.
385 And yif so be his hed be gret, than put to your hande; put hym in ayen and a-noynt the mouthe [f. 13v] of the matrice with softe onymentis, as oyle of olyue or laury, and lete the mydwyf wete here handis in watir of senigreue that lyne-seede hath be soden in, and than sese the hed and drawe hym forth.
390

And yif the child lyth a-'yens' kende, than let the moodir lye on an harde bed, so that she haue hir hed and hir shuldris esily leyd an hye, and than wysely put to your hand and dresse so that he may come foorth in due maner and so drawe hym foorth and ese
395 tymely the woman.
And yif he hold with the too hand, loke ye drawe hym not forth, for so ye myght disioynt hym; but set youre fyngris on his shuldris and put hym in a-yen and dresse his handis to his sydis, and than take hym be the hed and drawe hym foorth. And yif he holde oute
400 bothe his handis, put your 'on' hand on his to shuldir and your

377 Now ... childe] om. S   383 dysioynted] S, disioyned C   384 his] the S
385 hande] + & S   387 laury] lawryne S   391 kende] + that is when he commethe
furthe hes face loking vp to hes mothers face S   392 an] and S   she] + may S
393 an] & S   400 on] to S

scholdyre & yowur othere [f. 15] hande on þe oþer scholdyre, &
dresse a-vysydly hys hondys to hys sydys & þen by þe hede drav
hym forth & be þe handys.

 And yf he schew hys fete & þe remmenavnt a-byde with-in,
405 mys-turnyde with-in þe matrice, put to yowur hande & dresse hym
as I have ofte sayde a-fore & sese hym by þe fete & draw hym so
forth.

 And yf he schew but hys oo legge, sese hym nevyre þan but put
to yowur honde to hys forkys & put hym a lytyll a-gaynne & seke
410 besyly þe oþer foote & yoyne hys fete to-gedyre &, yf ȝe mow, do
hys hondys to hys sydys & be þe fete so to drav hym forth. And yf
he dysyonne hys fete in commynge forth, put þat oo fote on þat oo
syde & put oþer on þat othyre syde, & put to yowur honde &
yoyne þe fete to-gethyre & dresse þe handys to þe syde & so draw
415 hym forth.

 And yf he schew hys hede & be turnyde on þat on syde or þat
oþer be-foore or [f. 15v] be-hynde, put to yowur hande & dresse
þe hand comen`a′bely & sese hym be þe scholdrys & so draw hym
forth a-vysydly & softly þat ye brysse not þe matryce.

420 And yf he schew hys kneys, put in yowur hand & so put hym in
a-gaynne and dresse hys hondys & tak hys fete & so tak hym
forth. And yf he schew hys bottok, put hym in a-gayne & dresse
hym as I seyde be-fore & so tak hym forth. And yf he schew hys
hede and hys fete yontly, put to yowur hande & display hym &
425 dresse hym so þat ye may tak hym owte by þe hede. There was a
chylde onys þat was takyn fro hys modere, hys handys & hys fete
yoynyde to-gedyrre, & both they lyuyd longe afture, but þe
modyre was long syk.

 And yf he have all hys membrys yoynyd to-gedyre or yf he ley
430 ouyrthwart, put to yowur hond & yf ye may any maner [f. 16]
dothe in þe forme as I have seyd be-forre: in wyche party of þe

401 yowur] the BA 402 a-vysydly] wisely BA 405 to] *om.* B 406 a-fore] *om.* B
409 hym] + inne B 410 mow] may B 411 to²] *om.* B 412 in] *om.* B þat oo¹] þe
oon B on] over B þat oo²] þe oon B 413 on] over B þat] þe B 417 be-hynde]
+ but D 419 a-vysydly & softly] softely B, wysly A brysse] brose BA 420 hand]
handis B   429 he²] + or yf he D   430 may] + by B   maner] + of wise B
431 be-forre] afore or B

other hand [f. 14] on the tother shuldre, and dresse wysely his handis to his sydis and than, be the hed and be the handes, drawe hym forth.

And yif he shewe his feet and the remanent a-byde with-jnne
405 a-mys, than is he turned in the matrice. Than put to your hand and dresse hym as I sey'd' be-fore; sese hym be the feet and drawe hym forth.

And yif he shewe but his on leg, sese hym neuer but put your hand to his fourches and put hym jn a litill a-yen and seke besyly
410 the tother foot and than joyne his feet to-gedir and, yif ye may, do his handis to his sydes and be the feet so drawe hym forth. And yif he disioyne his feet in comynge forth, than ley the to foot on 'þe' to syde and the tother foote on the tother syde, than put to your hand and ioyne the feet to-gedir and dresse his handis to his sydes
415 & drawe hym forth.

[f. 14v] And yif he shew his hed and be turned on the too syde or on the tother be-fore or be-hynde, put to your hand and dresse the hed comenable, and sese hym be the shuldris and drawe hym foorth.

420   And yif he shewe his knees, put to your hand and put hym a-yen, dresse his handis and sese his feet and so drawe hym foorth. And yif he shewe his buttok, put hym a-yen and dresse hym as I seyd be-fore and so take hym foorth. And yif he shewe hed and feet to-gedir, put to your hand and display hed and feet
425 a-sonder and dresse hym so that ye may take hym be the hed. Ther was onys a chyld take fro his moodir, hed and his feet joyned to-gedir, and both lyuyd longe aftir, but the moodir was longe syke.

And yif he haue all his membris ioyned to-gedir or if he be
430 ouer-thwert, put to your hand. And if ye may in any maner dresse hym and sese [hym] [f. 15] as I seide be-fore, be what part ye may

408 neuer] not S   put] + to S   409 besyly] *om.* S   411 and] + so S   so] *om.* S
413 to²] *om.* S   414 hand ... his] *om.* S   420 hym] + in S   422 buttok] buttokis S
hym] in S   426 moodir] + his S   his²] *om.* S   431 hym²] hem S, *om.* C

body ye may esyly se hym, holdyth hym & so tak hym forth. But euyre-more desyre to tak þe chylde by þe hede or ellys by þe fete, for tho be þe most [esyest] way of all.

435   And yf þer be mo than on chylde & yf þey schew hem yontly in þe nek of þe maˈtˈrys, with yowur hand put a-gaynne þe toon to þe oon syde & drawhith forth þat oþer. And aftyre take hym forth þat a-bode last.

Yf þe secundynne þat þe chylde lyth wrappydde in commyth
440 not forth with hym, than let þe mydwyffe help þe woman þat trauelyth & take þe secundynne on what part sche may & draw hit forth. And yf hit so be-fall þat hit be goon to þe bottvm of þe maˈtˈrys, sche þat ys delyuyrd, lett here forsse all [f. 16v] that sche can for-to put hyt forth & yf þe secundynne be holdon with þe
445 matryce, þan let þe mydwyffe draw hit forth a lytyll to þe on syde & a lytyll to þe oþyre. But lok þat sche draw not euyn forth, for þan myth sche lytely þer-with draw ovte þe matryce. And yf þe movth of þe matryce be so clos þat sche may not help in [with] hare hande, vse þan thyngis þat been wrytte heere-afture for þe
450 delyuerance of þe secundyn, for be þe help of þe[m], all þat þat ys stopyt schall out and all þat ys in þe matryce oþer than schold be of ryȝht, schall passe by þe medycyn.

Aftere þat þe chylde be borvnne, lok ȝe bynd hys navyll a lytyll fro þe wombe & a lytyll fro thens bynde hit with a-nothyre threde
455 so þat he blede not to moche. And whan he hath a lythyl restyde hym ovte of hys modere wombe, than let hys navyll be cutt in þys [f. 17] manere: ley hym vp-on a borde & aftyre tak with yowur to fyngyrs þat oon byndynge in yowur on hand & yowur oþer ij fyngyrs on þat oþer byndynge, & than with a rasere or a scharpe
460 knyffe kit þe navyll by-twene both byndyngys. And assentyth nevyre to þe foly of sume olde women þat were wont to kot hym

---

432 body] + þat B   esyly … hym] sease hym esily B   holdyth … forth] *om.* B; + & doth in þe maner as I have sayde a-fore, or in þe wyche party of þe body ye may se hym essely D   434 esyest] B, esely D, esy A   way] weyes B   443 sche … delyuyrd] *om.* B   forsse] + hir BA   444 can] may BA   445 forth] softe BA   446 oþyre] + syde BA   448 with] B, *om.* D   450 þem] þe D, thoo B, þo A   451–52 schold … of] *om.* B   454 thens] the ende B   459 a²] *om.* B   460 both] the 2 B, þe A

esyli, and whan ye haue hym dressid, wysely take hym forth and euer more desire to take hym be the hed or be the feet, for tho are most esy.

435 And yif ther is mo than oo childe and shewe hem in the necke of the matrice, than with your hand put a-yen the ton to the ton syde and drawe foorth the tother. And alwey be war and wys that ye dele and drawe softly for brosynge of the matrice.

Yif the secundyne that the chylde is wrappid in come not foorth 440 with hym, than let the mydwyf cache the secundyne on what part she may and drawe it foorth. And if so be that it be go to the botom of the matrice, than let the woman that is deliuered enforce hire-self in all that she may to put it foorth. And yif the secundyne be fastnyd or holden with the matrice, than let the mydwyf drawe 445 it softe a litill to the to syde and a litill to the tother syde, but [f. 15v] drawe it not even foorth, for thanne she myght lightly drawe oute the matrice. And yif the mouth of the matrice be so close that she may not helpe in with her hand, than vse these thynges that are wreten heer-aftir for deliueraunce of the 450 secundyne and all that is in the matrice other than it shuld be of right, it shal owte.

Affter the child is born, bynde his navill a litill fro the wombe and a litill fro thens bynde it with a-nothir threed so that he bleede 455 not to mech. And whan he hath a litill restid hym owte of his moodris wombe, than let his navill be cut on this wyse: ley it vpon a boord and than take with your too fyngris the to byndynge in your on hand and your other ij fyngres on the tother byndynge, and than with a rasour or a sharpe knyf cut the navill betwen the 460 byndynges. And assent ye neuer to the foly of summe old women that were wonte to cut them with glas or with a pece of an erthen

433 tho] they S   438 dele and] *om.* S   445 softe a litill] softly S   448 in] *om.* S
458 on hand and] handis S   459 and] *om.* S   461 with²] *om.* S

with glas or with a pese of a potte of erthe or with a scharp ston,
or all þat ys but foly & wyche-crafte.

And viij or x ovyre aftyre the chylde ys borvne, þan ȝyff hym
465 mete at þe bygynnynge þat may purge hys stomak & hys wombe
& norsch þe chylde, as ys hony a lytyll sodyn, for & yf hit be raw
hit schall mak hym svell & yf hit be ouer-moche sodyn hit schall
bynde hys wombe & hys stomak. Thus schall yow fede hym: wete
yowur fyngyre in þe hony & put hit in to hys movth & let hym sok
470 hit wele & þan ȝyf hym mylk, [f. 17v] but lok ye gyve hym not
hys modyrs mylk [fyrst] for be-cause of þe travelynge þat sche
hath had & þe purgacyon, for þat mylk ys not so good and
holsame as oþer ne wyll not [defye] so lyȝthly as oþer tyll sche
have restyd a whylle; & svmme say þat hyt were good for a chyld
475 to drynk þe mylk of ix women be-fo`o´re he drank eny of hys
modere & þan hys modere mylk ys best for hym.

Tak a norse for hym to kepe þe chylde þat be yong & in good
stat, þat hath twyes trauelyd of chyld, þat be of good [color] &
hath large brestys & not to schort pappys & þat þe openynge of
480 them be not to wyde, & wel a-vysyd & not wrathfoll, & þat sche
lovyth þe chylde with all here hert ne þat sche be not dronklew of
ouer-moche drynk, but euer let here ete wele & lette here sume
tyme travayle þat sche fall not costyff. And þat sche entermet not
of dedeuyt [f. 18] of dewery, for of þat myȝght fall here
485 purgacyon & tak a-way here mylk & mak hym dry.

And lok ye do not afture svme old women þat gyf here norysse
to ete, when here mylk faylyth, þe estrayne of schepe or of kow or
of oþer bestys femalys for-to recovyre here mylk, & þat but
encomburth þe stomak þat hyt may not defy here mete & so hit
490 turnyth to corrupcion & rotyth þe chylde. And lok ye take suche a
norse þat hathe mylk sumdell whyte but not all pale ne semblabyll

463 all] *om.* B   466 as ... sodyn] and þat it be well seasoned B   &²] *om.* B   469 þe]
om. BA   470 mylk] + but lok ye gyue [f. 17v] hym mylk D   471 fyrst] first B,
fryrst D   travelynge] travell B   þat] *om.* B   472 & ... purgacyon] *om.* B   good
and] *om.* BA   473 defye] B, defyed D   lyȝthly] sone B   474 þat] *om.* BA
475 be-fo`o´re] + þat B   476 modere¹] moders mylke BA   477 to ... chylde] *om.* B
478 chyld] + and BA   þat²] + she BA   color] colour B, calor D   482 here¹] *om.* B
ete] hete B   483–84 not ... dewery] hyr not with man B   here] + to B   485 hym]
hem B   486 ye do] *om.* B   487 estrayne] vddernesse B   of²] + a B   491 but] ne B

pott or with a sharp ston, [f. 16] ffor all these are foly and wichcrafte.

And the viij or the x howr after the child is born, gyf hym mete
465 at the begynnynge that may purge his stomak and his wombe and norysh, as is hony a litill sodyn, for yif [it] be raw it will make to swelle and yif it be ouer-mech soden it will bynde his wombe and his stomak. Thus shal ye feede hym: weete your fyngris in 'þe' hony and put it to his mowth and lete hym sowke it wel and than
470 gif hym mylke but not of his mooder firste, be-cause of here traueylynge, for that mylke is not so holsum to hym at the firste as othir woman mylke is, nor wil not so sone purge hym and defye in his stomak, till the woman haue restid here a while. And summe men sey that it were good for a child to sowke mylke of ix women
475 afore his moodris mylk and aftir þat his moodris mylke is beste to hym.

Yiff ye take a norys to your child, se that she be yonge and in good state, [f. 16v] that hath trauailed twyes of chyld, and that she be of good colour and haue large brestis and not 'to' short pappis
480 and that the openyng of them be not 'to' large. And that she [be] wyse and wel avised and not angry nor wrathfull. And that she loue the chyld and that she loue to ete and drynke wel clenly and that she dispose here so that she falle not costyf. And that she vse not her body with man, for that myght falle to take a-wey here
485 mylke.

And lok ye do not aftir summe olde women that yeue norcis, whan here mylke failith, to ete the estreen of sheep or of cow or of othir femell bestis, to recouer her mylk; and encombrith here stomak that she may not defie her mete and so turnyth to
490 corrupcion and hurtith the child. And see the norce haue mylke sumdel whyte and not pale, and that it be not thenne but sumdel

462 with] *om.* S   foly] but folyshe S   464 the²] *om.* S   465 purge] + hime S
466 it¹] S, *om.* C   make] + hem S   468 hym] + ye Shall S   fyngris] finger S
469 to] in S   470-71 firste ... firste] ffor that is not so holsum at the firste tyme for her
travellyng as S   473-76 And ... hym] *om.* S   478 that¹] + she S   480 be²] S, by C
482 wel] + & S   487 failith] is nere gonne S   ete] *om.* S   of²] + a S   488 mylk]
+ agyne S   490 child] + & so the nvrse have no mylke S   And] But S   the²] your S
491 not¹] no thinge S   sumdel²] som what S

to þat, & þat hit ʻbeʼ not to thyn but sumdell thyk, þat an ye put hit
on yowur hande hit rynnyth not lythely dovne & a party
droppynge lytyll be lytyll, for suche mylk ys good & most
495 holsome & norschynge þe chylde.

Yf þe modere whyle sche was with chylde was euer in good
poynt & delyueryde [at] conueniant tyme & yf þe chylde have all
hys membrys ryȝght as he schold have, & all þe [pores] and
[f. 18v] oþer openyng of hys body be large, & yf he had a stronge
500 woyce whan he comme fyrst fro hys modere, & yf a man towche
hym on eny party of hym þat he bray a-now, all þes be synnes þat
he ys lyfly and borvne in a commenabill tyme & esy to norche.
There her lytyll holys full on a mannys body & womannys, not so
gret as þe poynt of a nedyll, be the whyche swet got ovte of a man
505 & of a woman & þey been powrys.

How ye schall kepe þe chylde þe fyrst yere. Let hym be wasch
euery day onys or ellys tweys & nonne oftyre but more [myster]
be, for ofte bathynge or waschynge schall do hys hede harme; but
let þe norse gyfe hym mylk ofte on þe day, now at þe oon bryste
510 & now oon þat oþer, for þe chylde ys not of povyre to draw of þe
oon brest all þat hym nedyth, & þerfor as ofte as sche knowyth þat
he hath talent, gyve hym sok. But a-vyse yow wele he sok not
[f. 19] a-noon be-foore he ys bathyd ne in hys bathynge, for yf he
do, hyt schall do mvche harme at hys hert, for wete ye wyle þat þe
515 chyld þat is bathyd in any of [þo] tymes schall have dyuerse
sekenes þe tyme of hys lyffe, & lok þat he be in good eyere &
fede hym whan he ys mery & þan schall nonne corrupcyon hym
greve ne entyre with-in hym but þat he schall cast hyt vp a-gayne
sonne.
520 How & whan þe chylde bc veynd. Whan he ys of age of j yere
or ij, so þat he have tethe þat he may ete dyuerse metys, than vse
hym fro þe bryst; & a lytyll be-foore, yef hym softe metys & svete

491–92 semblabyll … &] all whyte ne B   494 mylk] *twice* D   495 holsome]
holsummest B   497 at] B, & D   conueniant] conuenable B   498 pores] poorys B,
pore D   501 bray] crye B   a-now] anoon B   502 lyfly and] lawfully B   505 & of]
or B   been] + called B   507 ellys] *om.* B   nonne] no B   oftyre] more B   but]
+ þe B   myster] B, mystery D   510 oon þat] at þe B   512 wele] + þat B   515 þo]
tho B, þe D   516 þat] *om.* B   520 ofʼ] + þe B   521 or] + of B   522 bryst] brestis B

thykke, that and ye put in your hand it renne not lyghtly down, but a party droppynge be lityll and be litill. [f. 17] Ffor suche mylke is good and moste holsum and norishynge.

495

And yif the mooder whil she was with child was alwey in good poynte and deliuerid at tyme, and if the child haue all his membris right as he shuld haue, and that the pooris and other [openynges] of his body be large, and yif he had a stronge voys whan he come
500 ferste forth of his moder, and yif a man twyk hym be any part that than he crye, all these ar signes that he is lyfly and born at comenabill tyme, and esy to norce.

505

How ye shal kepe the child the firste yeer. Lete hym euery day be washe onys or twyes and non oftener but more nede be, for ofte bathynge and washynge will hurte his hed, but lete his norce yeue hym mylke often on the day, now on the ton breste, now on the
510 tother, for the child is not of power to drawe on the ton breste that he nedith; and be war that he sowke not a-non before [f. 17v] his bathynge nor in his bathynge, for if he do, it shal harme hym at his herte. Therfore yif ye so do, it shal turne to diuers syknesses terme of his lyf. And loke that he be in good eyre and fed whan he is
515 mery and than shal no corrupcion greve hym nor entre hym, but he shal sone [caste] a-yen.

520 How ye shal wene your child: whan he is oon yer of age or ij, so that he hath teeth that he may ete diuers metis, than vse fro the brestis and a litill a-fore gyf hym softe metis and sweet and be

493 and be litill] *om.* S   494 norishynge] noryshethe best S   496 yif] *om.* S   the ... she] while the mother S   child] + she S   497 at] + good S   498 openynges] openyngis S, openenynges C   499 come] came S   500 a ... twyk] one touche S 501 than] *om.* S   502 comenabill] convenient S   506-07 euery ... be] *om.* S 507 more] *om.* S   508 his hed] hem S   509 breste] + & S   512 nor ... bathynge] *om.* S   513 so do] *tr.* S   514 fed] fede hem S   515 entre] + in S   516 caste] S, taste C   521 vse] + hem S

for-to ete & be lytyll and lytyll draw þe tete fro hym, & at þe last
anoynt þe tetys ende with some bytter þynge & lothly, so þat hyt
525 may loth hym & for'y'ete hys sokynge; yf þe norse be to
habvndant of mylk, let put here to gret labore of body so þat be
labor sche [f. 19v] may [be] a-swagyd, & let euery norse be ware
þat sche ete no salt metys & byttyre, for þat schall rot þe schylde
or he comme to eny gret age.
530   And seth here be-forre I have told yow what suffocacyon &
precypytacion been & where-of þey comme, now woll I tell yow
þe sygnes þat ye schall know þat oon fro þe oþer and than wyll I
tell yow þe synes of all þe euyls of þe matryce. The sygnes of
suffocacyon of marys ben þes: yf sche draw here breth with
535 dyffyculte & schortly & lythyll, for þan þe matrys rysyth to þe
hert, [hyr iointis, hyr handis, hir feet, her brestys] been sore &
suellynge a-bowte here hert, here wyket ys more fat þan hyt was
wont to be, þe waynes of here front ryson & svellyn, a cold swete
rysyth on here face & be here hede, here [powls] [steryth] but
540 lythyll. Othyrwhyle þe paynne commyth ofte & passyth sonne.
And oþer-whyll þey wene hit be þe govte. But þer ys dyuersyte
by-twene þe gowt and [f. 20] þat, for sche þat hathe þe gowte,
mochyll spetyll schall a-ryse in here movth & þere passe, but here
matrys a-bydyth stylle in here place. And þe suffocacyon makyth
545 þe matryce to a-ryse to þe hert & hare pulse ys styll & no spetyll
commyth oute & makyth here to swoune & makyth here also to
covrbe to-gedyre here hede & hare kneys.
         Whan þeys thyngis fall to a woman, let cowche here in a fayre
bedde & hote so þat hare hede be hy, as hytt were in syttynge, &
550 þan anoynt here with oyle lavryon & frot wele hare hondys & hare
fete & tak a fethyre & wet hit in hott watere & wete well here face
þer-with & makyth hote [yower] hondys & chaf well here brystys

523 tete] tetis B   526 let] + hir B   so] *om.* BA   527 be¹] BA, *om.* D   528 no] not
over B   529 or] + þat B   530 here] *om.* B   532 þat²] the B   wyll I] I woll B
534 marys] the matrice B   536 hyr¹ ... brestys] B, *om.* D   537 here wyket] the
mowthe of her wombe B   fat] fatter B   539 rysyth] rennyth B   powls] B, pourys D
steryth] stirreth B, steryd D   541 govte] + kynde B   543 þere] þus B   545 to¹] *om.* B
545–46 no ... commyth] maketh no spatylle B   swoune] swete B   548 in] on BA
549 & ... hy] *om.* B   550 þan] let B   550–52 &² ... hondys] *om.* B   552 yower] you
D

litill and litill drawe the breste fro hym, and than a-noynte the
pappis with sum bitter thynge so þat he may lothe and forsake his
525 sowkynge. Yif the norce be 'to' habundaunte of mylk, let put here
to gret labour of body so that be labour she may a-swage, and
ware euery norce that she ete no salte metis and bitter, for tho will
rote the child or he come to any gret age.

530 [f. 18] Heere ye shal knowe of diuers siknesses that were spoke
of a-fore, that is [to] seyn, suffocacion an precipitacion of þe
matrice, and wherof thei come, and the signes to knowe the ton fro
the tother, and all the euyll of the matrice. Signes of suffocacion
of the matrice ar these: yif she drawe hire breth with difficulte and
535 shortly and litill, thanne the matrice risith toward hire herte, and
than her joyntis, hire handes, hir feet and here breest be [sore] and
swellyng a-bowte here herte, here priuite is more fat than it was
wonte to be, the veynes of here front rysen and swellen, a cold
swet rysit ouer here face and here hed, and here pouce sterith but
540 litill. Othirwhile the peyne comyth often and passith sone, and so
thei wene it were the gowte; mechill spatill risith in here mouth
and there passith, but the matrice bidith stille in here place. And
suffocacion makith [f. 18v] the matrice to ryse to the herte, hir
pouce is stille and no spatill comyth owte and it makith hire to
545 cowre to-gedir hir hed and her feet.

Medycines for suffocacion whan this dishese fallith to a
woman. Ley hir hote faire vpon a bed so that here hed be hye, [as]
550 it were in syttyng, and frete wel here handis and here feet, and
than a-noynte hem with oyle laurion and wete a fedir in hote watir
and wete wel here face ther-with and make hote your handys and

---

523 than] *om.* S   524 lothe] + them S   525 let] *om.* S   526 a-swage] + her mylke S
527 ware ... norce] lett euery nvrse beware S   metis] meat S   and] not S   tho]
they S   528 any] a S   531 to] S, *om.* C   an] or S   536 be sore and] *om.* S   sore]
fore C   542 there] + so S   but] and S   And] + 'yf' S   544 pouce is] pounccs are S
549 as] S, at C

& here wombe & meue ofte her chynne & put to hare nosse
thyngys of strong savore, as ys castory & galbanum & brent cloth
555 & fetherys bront. And be-nethe at here wyket lete hare tak a
fumygacyon of herbys or [f. 20v] spycys of good savore, as ys
lignum aloe, muske & cost & olyuys & make here a pessary of
[yrelyon], mustelyon, camelion, nardilion, for þes woll draw þe
sedys & þe flourys dovne. And yf sche be strong & not to febyll &
560 have eten lytyll, let here blode vndyre þe anckle of here fote &
ʒyff here to drynk þe siruppe of calamynt [&] yerapigra with þe
jusse of wormwode. & good ys to wasch here wyket with water
[þat] nepte or calament hath be soden yn. And [tak] dry comyn &
stampe hit & gyffe here to drynk. Or for-to tak þe grece of a fox or
565 þe sewet of a gotte & medyll hit with aspaltum & put hit in with a
pessary. Aftyre tak þe rote of holyhock, wylde malov & flex &
lynsed & stampe hem to-gythyre & wrynge owte þe juce & chaffe
here wyket þer-with & þat plaster ys good layde to here navyll.
And yf hit so be here matrys go to hy whan sche hath chyldydde,
570 let hare parch otys in a panne & mak hem hote & as [f. 21] hote as
sche may suffyre, put hem in a bagge & bynde hem to here
wombe.

    A good drynk for þe suffocacyon. Tak þe sede of netlys &
stampe hem to poudyre & gyffe hem to drynk in wynne & sche
575 schall be holpon a-nonne. And yf hare speche fayle & be in parell
of dethe & sche may not reseyve no drynk, tak grene rew & frot
hit well be-twene yower handys & put hit in-to here noosse; or tak
aspaltum & ley hit vp-on quyck colys & put hit to here nosse. And
yf ye se þat sche be in gret parell of dethe, tempyre castoryum in
580 wynne & put hit in here movth. A stermuntacyon for þe same
evyll. Take fethyr-wort with j ʒ, j drame castorium j ʒ, tak thes &
put þem [powdered] in here nosse.

---

555 here wyket] the mowthe of her wombe B   556 or] + of B   557 here] *om.* B
558 yrelyon] vrelyon D, vrelioun B   559 to] *om.* BA   560 lytyll] *om.* BA   561 þe¹]
om. B   &] B, or D   562 &] + it B   here wyket] the mowthe of hir wombe B
563 þat] BA, of D   And] Also B   tak] B, for-to D   564 grece] + oute B
565 aspaltum] a spalter B   566 malov] malowes B   568 here wyket] the mowth of
her wombe B   layde] to ley B   569 be] + that BA   574 hem²] hir BA   576 not]
om. B   579 of dethe] *om.* B   581 j¹ … drame] *om.* B   castorium] + ana B
582 powdered] B, poudyre D   nosse] nosethryllis B

chafe wel here brestis and hire wombe and meve ofte her chyn and
put [to] her nose thyng of stronge savour, as castori & galbanum
555 and brent cloth or brent ffederis. And be-nethe at here priuite lete
hire [haue] a suffumigacion of spicis or erbis of good savour, as
lignum aloe, muste and softe of oliues and make here a pissarye of
[yrelion], mostelion, [f. 19] camelys, nardileo, for thes will drawe
the sedis and the floures down. And if she [be] stronge and not
560 febill and haue etyn, lete here bloode vnder the ankyll of hire
foote and gif here drynke sirip of calamynte, or gerapigra with the
jus of wormood, and good it is to wash here priuite with watir that
nepte or calamynte hath be sodyn in. And to [take] drye comyn
and stampe it and yeue here to drynke, or to take the gres of a fox
565 or the suet of a got and medyll it with [aspalte] and put it in with a
pissary.

570

A good drynke for suffocacion. Tak the seed of nettill and
stampe hem to powder and yeue here to drynke in wyn and she
575 shal haue helpe a-non. And if here speche faile and be in perel of
deth and may not reseyf drynke, than tak grene rue and frete it wel
be-twen your handis and put to here nose. Or take [aspaltum] and
ley it on qwyk [f. 19v] colis and put to here nose. And if she be in
gret perel of deth, than tempir castorium in wyn and put it in here
580 mouth. A stermutacion for the same. Take fethirwort, wey3te j 3,
de struccion j 3, of castorium j 3, stampe thes thynges, put them to
ther nase therlys.

---

554 to her nose] some S   galbanum] + or assa fetida S   555 and] or S
555-56 be-nethe ... suffumigacion] lett her have a fumygacyon benethe at her previtte S
556 haue] *om.* C; *cf.* S   557 muste] + i.e. vinygre *above line* S   and ... olives] *om.* S
558 yrelion] vrelion C   558-59 yrelion ... down] the same with woll S   559 be]
om. CS   560 and ... etyn] *om.* S   561 here] + to S   563 or] & S   take] S, *om.* C
564 to^2] *om.* S   565 aspalte] S, aspale C   574 yeue] + it S   577 put] + it S
aspaltum] S, aspartum C   578 put] + it S   580-82 A ... therlys] *om.* S

The sygnes how ye schall know whan þe matrys ys remewydde
of hys ryȝth plase: gret angysch & paynn ys þer a-bouth, & but
585   helpe be þe sonere doon, many wondys & grevys & chynnys schal
rysse in þe matrysse. [f. 21v] And whan he rysyth so hy þat hit
comme to þe hert & oppressyth so, as I have sayde here be-for, þat
sche ys well ny strangelyde & vom commyth & spetyll as eysell &
þe movthe full of watyre & here hede & here tonge quakyn & hare
590   speche ys lost, tak a pynne & bynde hit a-bovthe with woll thyck
& than wet hit in oyle de [bavme] or ony oþer oyle of good savor
& put hit in at here wyket & tak aspaltum & put hit [to] here
noosse, or ellys þe horne of a got or þe legge of a deere brent, or
fethyrs brent, & wete hit in vynegere & hold hit to here nosse.
595   And yf sche may opynne here mowth & spek, gyue hare castorium
in wynne & wete yowur fyngers in oyle & hold hit to hare nose,
but tak not þe pynne a-way with [þe] woll tyll sche be hole, for yf
sche be opyn beneth þe euyll woll comme a-gaynne. And yf þe
matrice be fallyn donward, þes be þe synes: sche schall have
600   stronge [dysesse] in here bladdyre, hare leggis quakyn, here vryne
ys stopyd: [f. 22] doth þan þe medycyn of precipitacion.

Yf a woman have to muche of hare flourys, yf hit comme of
blode, þan let hare blode in hare harme on þe vayne epatik or on
þe hond, for-to draw þe blode vpwarde, for hit will rynne euer
605   more & draw thedyre as hit hath yssev. Good ys to set a ventosse
by-twene hare pappys. And yf hit comme of blode, tak þe juce of
plantayne & lay þer-in thosydde woll of þe front of a scheppe &
put hit in at here wyket well depe. Or ȝif here to drynk þe juce of
syngrene with rede wynne or tak [wolle] & wet hit in þe juce &
610   lay hit to hare navyll. Also tak þe [rote] of þe red dok and seth hit
in wynne or watyrre & ȝiff here to drynk. Also thyngis þat been
cold is good to here to vse.

584 ryȝth] grett B   paynn] akyng BA   585 sonere] sone B   586 he] hit BA   hit]
he B   588 vom] foome B, womyth A   589 quakyn] quakyng B   hare] the B
591 bavme] bayme D, baune B   ony] in BA   592 at … wyket] in the mowthe of her
wombe B   to] BA, *om.* D   595 opynne] *twice* D   597 þe²] BA, *om.* D   598 sche]
it B   600 dysesse] dissease B, dycsse D   here¹] *om.* B   quakyn] quakyng B
603 in] on BA   605 yssev] + And BA   607 a] the B   608 here wyket] þe mowthe of
hir wombe B   609 or] to B   wolle] BA, wlle D   610 rote] B, rose D   þe²] *om.* B
611 thyngis] thyng BA   þat] *om.* B

The signes that ye shal knowe whan the matrice is remeved oute of right place: she felith gret angwish and akyng ther a-bowte, and
585 but if helpe be the sunner, many woundes and grevous chynnes shal rise in the matrice and whan it risith hie toward the herte, it inpressith it so sore, as I seide be-fore, that she is ner strangelid and vomet comyth and spatill as eysel and here mowth full of watir, hir hed and her tunge quakyn and hir speche is lost. For this
590 dishese take a penne and bynde it a-bowte thykke with wulle and than wete it in oyle of bawme or in other of good savour and put it in here priuite. [f. 20] And take aspale (mole) and put to here nose or the horn of a got or the leg of a der brent or federis, and wete in vyneger and hold it to here nose and if she may open here mouth
595 and speke, gif here castorium in wyne and wete your fyngris in oyle and hold to here nose, but take not the penne with wulle till she be hol, for yif she be openyd be-nethe the euil will come a-yen. And yif the matrice be falle dounward, thes are the signes: she shal haue stronge dishese in hire bladdere, hir leggis qwakyn,
600 hire vryn stoppid; do than the medicines of precipitacion afore seid.

And yif it come of blood, than let here blood on hir arme on the veyne epatyk or on the hand to drawe the blood vpward, for it will renne euer more thedir as it hath jssew. And good it is to set a
605 ventouse be-twen her pappys. [f. 20v] Medicines for the matrice fallen dounward, yif it come of blood. Tak juce of playnteyn and ley theron faire tosid wulle of the fronte of a shep and put it in at here priuite wel and deepe, or gif here drynke juce of senigrene with red wyn and wete wolle in the jus therof and ley it to here
610 navyll. Also take the rote of red docke and sethe it in wyn or in watir and gif hir to drynke. Alle thynge that is cold is good for here to vse.

584 right] hes S   585 if] *om.* S   589 quakyn] quakynge S   591 it] + wulle and than wete C   592 in] + to S   And] *om.* S   592-93 aspale ... or] *om.* S   593 wete] + it S 600 stoppid] stoppethe S   606 fallen] fallinge S   607 at] *om.* S   608 or] & S   gif] make S   senigrene] fengreue S   609 wete] + this S   610 navyll] + & S 611 thynge] thengis S   cold] + for that S

And ȝif hit comme of colore, þat it ys good to geve here
laxatiuis, as ys trifera saraseta, sirup de violet & suche othyre
615 laxatiuis. And ȝif hit comme of habundance of flevme, tak
yeralogodyon & polipodin [f. 22v] & seth hit in wynne or in [ale]
& gyffe here to drynk. And whan þe body ys well clensydde of
euyll humors, þan ȝif here medycynys þat will strayne þe blode
with-inforth & let bath here in luck-warme water in wyche ben
620 sodyn rosys eglente, þe croppys of þe rede bryere, agrimony &
plantayne. And than aftere let a man ȝif hare straynabill drynkes,
as ys poudyre of corall, þe sede of folefote, pome granat, povdyre
of hertis horne, plantayn, centynody, sandragon; all þes ben good
to-gythyre or els eche by hym-selfe.
625 And good ys to drynk ptisan made with barly dryed be-fore &
sodyn in watyre. And whan hit ys cold, put a lytyll vynegyre & yf
þerto [ther be] sodyn plantayne with þe rotis þer-in, so muche þe
better. And it ys good for hyre to drynk water þat benys be sod in.
Or tak whete-melle & sethe hit with mylk or with hony & bynd hit
630 to here navyll. Or tak schepis [f. 23] donge or gresse of a gosse or
of a capon & stompe hit to-gythyre & mak a plastre.
An-oþer medycyn: tak egge scalys þat þe chekkys be [hacched]
in & mak poudyre þer-of, & gyffe þe woman drynk iij dayes
þer-of, as moche as sche may tak vp with here thumbe & hare to
635 fyngers, with cold watere.
An-oþer medycyn well [prouyd]. Tak a tode & bryn here in a
potte & tak of þat poudyre & put in a purse & honge hit a-bout
hare mydyll & be þe grace of God the cowrs schall sone seesse.
And ȝif ye woll preve hit, tak & hange þat poudyre a-bouth a
640 hennys nek to dayes by-forre ye sle here & þan draw of hare hede
& sche schall not blede. Or tak lynsed & as moche darnell & mak
poudyre of hem & ete hit at morvne & at eue with chese of a gote.
And yf þe flourys comme to surfetusly, tak vynys & brynne hem
to poudyre & put hem in a lynyn bagge & put hit in at here wyket.

614–15 as ... laxatiuis] *om.* B   tak] *om.* B   616 ale] BA, alle D   621 than] *om.* BA
aftere] + þat B   625 good] + it B   ptisan] a tissan B   dryed] drye B   626–27 & ...
be] & yf þerto D, therto and if ther be B   630 or¹] and B   632 scalys] shalys B,
schellys A   hacched] B, heget A, havtydde D   634 þer-of] + eche day B   vp] *om.* B
636 prouyd] proued B, prouoyd D   637 put] + hit BA   hit] *om.* B   640 by-forre]
+ or B   641 &²] or B   644 at ... wyket] the mowthe of her wombe B

And yif it come of colour, than gif her laxatiffis, as is trifera serracyneise, ebrose, sirep of violet and other suche laxatifiis. And
615 yif it come of habundans of flewme, than tak geralagodion and polipodium, that is fern that growith on an ok, and sethe it in wyn or in ale and gyf here to drynke. And whanne the body is wel clensid of euel humours, than gyf here medicynes that will streyne the blood with-jnfoorth. Medicynes to streyne the blood: lete
620 bathe here in [f. 21] lewke watir in which be sothen rosis eglentyn, croppis of the red brere, egrimony and plaunteyn. Than aftir that gyf here streynabill drynkis and powdir of corall, seed of fole-fote, pomegarnet, powdir of hertis horn, plauntyn, centinodye, sandregragon; all thes ar good to-gedir, or ellis ech be hem-silf.
625 And good is to drynke tysanys mad with barly dried a-fore and sothen in watir, and whan it is cold put a litill vyneger ther-to and yif planteyn with the rotys be sothyn þer-jn, it is the bettir. Also it is good to drynke the watir that benys haue be sodyn in. Or take whete-mele and sethe it with mylke or with hony and bynde it to
630 here nauyll. Or take shepis donge and goos gres or capons grece and stampe hem to-gedir and make a plastir.
Also tak egge shellis that chekens ar hacchid in and make powdir ther-of. [f. 21v] And gyf here [to] drynke thre dayes, eche day as meche as she may take vp at onys with here thombe and
635 hire iij fyngres with cold watir.
Also anothir medicyn wel provyd: take a tode and brenne hire in a pot to poudir, and take of that poudir and put it in a purs and hange it a-bowte here myddill and be the grace of God the cource shal sone sece. And yif ye will proue it, hange this powdir a-bowte
640 a hennys necke ij dayes er ye sle hir and drawe of here hed and she shal not bleede. Or take lynseed and as mech darnell and make powdir of them and ete it morwe and eve with chese of a gott. And if the ffloures come surfetously tak vynes and brenne hem to powdir and put hem in a lynen bagge and so put hem in-to here

---

613-14 as .... laxatiffis] *om.* S   615 and] *twice* C   616 that ... ok] *om.* S   620 lewke] + warme S   which] + hathe S   621 red brere] brynt S   625 good is] vse S   a-fore] *om.* S   627 yif] *om.* S   with] + yff S   630 and] or S   633 to] S, do C   635 iij] *om.* S   636 hire] hem S   639 sone sece] *tr.* S   639-41 And ... bleede] *om.* S   642 morwe] mornyg S   eve] evenynge S   644 in-to] in S

645   And yf hit comme be-[cause] [f. 23v] hyre matryce ys hurt for
cause of trauelynge of chylde, tak oyle iiij ʒ & medyll hit with old
butter & mak a pessary þer-of & put hit in & hit schall do gret
esse. ʒiff hit comme to surfetysly, tak horsdonge & tempyre hit
with wyneegyre &, as hote as sche may suffure hit, bynde hit to
650 here navyll & whan hit ys cold, het hit a-gayne & ley hit þer-to
more. Or tak þe here of hare hede & bynde hit a-bowte a grene tre,
what tre ye will, & hit schall stanche. Or tak black poppy &
poudyre made of þe scalys of eggys þat þe hen hath soton &
[fayllyd] of hare chykyn, & ʒiff here to drynk in wynne. Or sethe
655 lynsed, plantayne, & red nethyll in wynne & ʒiff hare [to] drynk.
Or tak þe rote of a herbe þat ys callyd comfyry & scrapp hit clene
& seth hit well in a nev pott of erthe in wynne & ʒif hare to drynk
iij dayes þer-of.
   ʒiff ye will change þe cowrs of þe flourys of eny woman in-to
660 oþer dayes, tak vij levys of þe fygge [f. 24] tre & stompe hem &
gyff hare to drynk in wynne & here covrs schall chavnge in-to
oþer dayes.
   Now syth I have told yow þe medycyns for superfluite of
flourys, now will I tell yow medycyns for þe retencion or faylynge
665 of flowrys, as whanne a woman hath nonne or ryʒht few. [B]vt yf
ye woll vndyrtak for-to mak þe flowrys of eny woman to comme,
ye muste fyrst vse þys medycyn viij dayes be-fore þe day & þe
tyme þat sche was wonte to have hare flowrys, of þe wyche ye
must be certayne of here-selfe. Tak a gret quantite of nepte & not
670 so moche of [sclarye] & þe myddyll rynde of chery tre, savayne,
betayne a lytyll quantite, boyle all þeys to-gythyre in whytte
wynne. And þe fyrst day of viij dayes be-fore hare tymme let hare
drynk j tyme. And þe ij day ij tymes & þe iij day iij tymes & so
euery day more and more to þe day of hare purgacyon. & [f. 24v]
675 mak a bath of heyhow, nepte, pulioll ryall, savayne, & let bath

645 be-cause] by cause B, be D   646 for cause] *om.* B   648 to] *om.* B   653 scalys]
shalys B, schellys A   soton] sytten B   654 fayllyd] fayled B, fallyd D   655 red]
þe B, *om.* A   to] BA, do D   656 þe ... of] *om.* B   660 hem] *om.* B   665 woman]
þei B   666 eny] *om.* B   667 day & þe] *om.* B   669 certayne] certified BA   of¹]
by B   670 sclarye] sclarye A, salarye B, *lacuna* D   of²] + þe B   671 all] *om.* BA
672 of] + the B   hare] the B   tymme] terme B   675 heyhow] horehounde B   ryall]
& BA

645 priuite. And yif thei come be-cawse hire matrice be hurte of
trauelynge of child, take oyle iiij ʒ and medill it with olde [f. 22]
butter and make a pissary therof & put in at here priuite and it shal
do here gret ese. Also take hors dunge and tempir it with vinegir
and, as hot as she may suffre, bynde it to here navyll and whan it
650 is cold hete it a-yen and ley it ther-to. Or take the her of hire hed
and bynde it a-bowte a grene tree, what tree ye will, and it shal
staunche. Or take blake popy and the poudir made of egge shellis
that the henne hath setyn and faylid of here checons, and gyf here
to drynke. Or tak the rote [of] camfory and scrape it well and sethe
655 it in a new pot of erthe in wyn and gyf here drynke iij dayes
therof. Or sethe lyne-seed, planteyn and nettill croppis in wyn and
gyf here.

Yiff ye will chaunge the cours of floures of a woman in-to other
660 dayes, take vij leuis of the fygge tree and stampe hem and gyf here
to drynk in wyn and þe cours shal chaunge in to other dayes.

[f. 22v] Medicines for retencion or failyng of floures. Whan a
woman hath non or ellis right fewe, yif ye will vndertake to make
665 the floures to come, ye muste firste vse these medicynes viij dayes
a-fore the day and the tyme þat she was wonte to haue the flouris,
of the which ye muste be certified be hire-self. Than take a gret
quantite of nepte and not so meche of clary and the myddilbark of
cheritre, saveyn, beteyn a litill quantite, and boyle these wel
670 to-gedir in white wyn. And the firste day of the viij dayes be-fore
here terme lete hire drynke on tyme, and the secunday ij tymes,
the thirday iij tymes, and so eueryday more and more to the tyme
of hire purgacion, and make a bath of heyhofe, nepte, puliall ryall
and saveyne and lete here bathe euery day fastynge. [f. 23] And
675 after mete or she go to sleep, make here a stue: let boyle 'wel' in a

645 be-cawse] + that S   649 suffre] + it S   650-52 Or ... staunche] *om.* S   653 the ...
checons] chekens hathe be hatched of S   654 tak] *om.* S   of] S, *om.* C   655-56 iij ...
therof] therof thre dayes S   657 gyf] + it S   659 Yiff ye] This S   a woman]
women S   664 right] very S   665 medicynes] + folowenge S   666 the flouris]
then S   667 of] *om.* S   671 terme] tyme S   tymes] + & S   675 let] *om.* S

hare euery day fastynge & aftyre mete, or sche go to slepe, mak
hare suche a stew: let boyle well in a potte lorer, savayn, nepte &
dytayne & mak hare a subfumigacyon for-to receyue þe savor
þer-of at hare wyket vp to hare matryce, as warme as sche may
680 suffure hit. But whan þe terme of har purgacion ys passyd, cesyth
of all þes thyngis saue of þe drynk ye schall ȝeue harre [as] ye
have do [before hir purgacioun, and þen doo all thyngis as ye haue
doon] but yf sche be hole in þe men tyme, & þan sesyth of all
thyngis.

685   A-nothyre medycyn þat a lady of Salerne vsyde. Tak perytory,
malovys, calamynt & þe daysy & let stampe hem & wrynge out þe
juse of þe forseyde herbys. Afture tak fayere flowere of whete &
tempyre hit with þe juce of þe forseyde herbys & mak þer-of
oblayes or crispys & ȝif hare þe fyrst day vij, þe ij day v, þe iij day
690 iij, & sche schall purge hare a-nonne. [f. 25] And yf þe flowrys
comme to surfetusly, do þat medycyn to hire þat ys wryttyn
be-fore in þe receyt of stanchynge of þe flowrys, þe whyche he
puttyth to profyrre þe prefe of þe henne.

        Galyen sayth þat a woman þat hath lost hare flowrys schulde
695 blede vndyre harre ancle j day on þat j fote, anoþer on þat oþer
fote, mesurabely as sche may bere, for þe blode will euyre draw
thedyre as hit hath yssev, & so schall sche mak hit [to] draw
donward.

        A medycyn for þe same: tak horhownd & stamp hit & draw hit
700 þorow a cloth & ȝiff hare to drynk with white wynne & þat herbe
ys good to bath harre ynne. And hit ys good whyle hit ys grene to
stamp hit & ley hit vndyr hare navyll. Or ellys lett sethe hit in a
pot &, also hote as sche may suffyre hit, let hare sitte þer-ouyre &
receyue þe fume in-to hare matrycc, & look sche be well couyrde
705 with clothys all a-boute, þat þe fume may well be holdyn [f. 25v]
ynne so that nonne passe but vpward. Or tak xxxvj bayes of lorere

---

675-76 bath hare] *tr.* BA   676 day] *om.* B   678 dytayne] betayn B beteyn A
679 wyket] wekett B   681 as] B, *om.* D   682–83 before ... doon] B, *om.* D   687 of
... herbys] *om.* B   Afture] then B   689 oblayes] oxles B   691 to¹] *om.* B
692 be-fore] afore B   stanchynge] changyng B   þe³] *om.* B   693 puttyth] + before B
profyrre] *om.* B   694 flowrys] + a moneth BA   695 harre] the B   fote] *om.* B
anoþer] + day BA   696 may] myght B   697 sche] ye B   to] B, do D   699 hit¹] the
juse B   703 also] as B   704 look] + þat B   well couyrde] *tr.* B   706 ynne] *om.* B

pot lorell, saveyn, nepte, beteyn and make hir a suffumygacion to
resseyue the sauour herof at hire priuite vp to here matrice, as
warme as she may suffre, and whan the terme of here purgacion is
paste, cesith of all thynges saf of the drynke that ye shuld gyf here
680 as ye did a-fore hire purgacion, than do all thynges as ye haue do,
but she be [hole] in menewhile, than cessith of all thynges.

685 Anodir medycyn that a lady Salerne vsid. Take peritory,
malwis, calamynte and the dayes-jees, stampe hem & wrynge
owte the juce, than take faire whete flour and tempir it with þe
juce and make ther-of oblees or crespes and gif hire the firste day
vij, the secunde day v, the third day iij, and [f. 23v] she shal purge
690 hire a-non. And yif the floures come to surfetously, than do the
medicyn to hire that is wreten a-fore in retencion of staunching of
floures, the whiche he puttith to preue the preef of them.

Galyon seith that a woman þat hath lost hire floures a monyth
695 shuld bleede vndir hir ankyll on day on the too foot, a-nother day
on the tother, mesurably as she myght bere, for the blood 'will'
drawe thedir as it hath jssew, and than shal she make it drawe
downward.
Take [hore hound] and stampe it, drawe oute the juce therof
700 throw a cloth and gyf hire to drynke with whight wyn and that
herbe is good to bathe hire jn, and it is good whill it is grene to
stampe and ley it vnder here navill, or ellis let sethe it in a pot and,
as hote as she may suffir, let hire syt therouer [f. 24] and receyue
the fume into here matrice, so that she be coueryd with clothes
705 a-bowte, that the fume be wel holden in so that non passe a-way.
Or take xxxvj^{ti} bayes of lorell and lete stampe hem in-to powdir

676 suffumygacion] fumygacion S   677 herof] benethe or S   678 suffre] + it S
679 paste] + and S   ye shuld] *tr.* S   680-81 than ... thynges] *om.* S   681 hole]
holde C   685 that ... vsid] *om.* S   686 dayes-jees] dayses juce S   689 and] + and C
691 in ... staunching] for restreynge S   692 the ... them] *om.* S   694 a monyth] *om.* S
695 hir] the S   696 myght] may S   697 she] ye S   699 hore hound] S, horond and C
it] + & S   oute ... therof] it S   702 it^1] *om.* S   let] *om.* S   703 suffir] + it S
therouer] ouer it S

and let stampe hem in-to povdyre & ȝif hare to drynck with whyte
wynne. Or tak saffron, galbanum & storak, of eche lyck moche,
þat ys to say half a vnce, & stamp hem to-gydyre & mak of hem
710   as hit werre a pessary & so vse hit.

And yf þe matryce be so hard þat hit hold þe flowyre þat hit
may not passe, tak lynsede & fenigrek, of ech j vnce, & temper
hem with hony & mak a pessary & vse hit. For-to mak þe flovrys
to come, all-thow þe matrys be out of hare ryȝht place, & for-to
715   mak a woman conceyve. Tak of botyr v ȝ, of juce of jsope 1 ȝ, of
myrre 1 ȝ, of þe sevet of a deere ij ȝ, of grece of a henne ij ȝ, of
terebentyne ij ȝ & of hony þat suffysyth; mak all þes [thyngis] to
sethe in a potte of erthe & vse hem as a pessary vndyrnethe. For
this pessary vsydde [Dame] Fabina Prycyll whan hare nature was
720   nygh wastydde, & sche [f. 26] was all hooll.

And are ye yeue hare eny medycyns, let hare vj or vij dayes
be-fore vse metys laxatyuys & drynkys & tak castorium &
tempyre hit with þe juce of pulioll & of calamynt & ȝiff hare to
drynk. Or tak pulioll & calamynt & sethe them in mede & þan dry
725   ham & mak poudyre of hem & of þat poudyre ȝif [hir] to drynk
with mede. [Dame] Cliopatre tavt þys medycyn to hare douter, ȝif
hare matryce were so induerde & hardyde þat hare flowrys myȝth
not passe. Sche bad tak þe gall of a boll or of a-noþer best, & þe
poudyre of myrre & þe juce of jsop, & methill hem to-gythere &
730   þan tak tosydde woll & mak a pessary þer-of & rolle hit & put hit
in so.

A-noþer: tak rwe, mynt, pulioll ryall, of eche lyche muche; iij
croppis of sauge, iij plantys of rede cole, iij hedys of lekys, &
sethe all þes in a pot of erthe with wynne & ȝif hare to drynk aftyr
735   hare bathynge. A-noþer: tak þe rote [f. 26v] of gladyoll & þe rote

707 let] bete & B   709 half a] *tr.* B   711 hard] harded BA   714 to] *om.* B   hare]
his BA   715 woman] + for to B   of¹] *om.* B   717 ij] an B, a A   thyngis] B,
tyngis D   to] and B   718 sethe] + hem B   vndyrnethe] *om.* B   719 pessary] *om.* B
Dame] BA, damd D   Prycyll] fabian porcille B, fabyan priciall A   721 are] if B
hare¹] *om.* B   hare²] + vse B   722 vse] *om.* B   metys … drynkys] mete & drynk
laxatyfe B   723 of¹] *om.* B   724 mede] methe B   dry] drynke B   725 hir] hem BA
to drynk] *om.*   726 Dame] BA, damd D   Cliopatre] thopar B   douter] + of hir
matrice B   728 of¹] *twice* D   729 myrre] + or of a-nutre A   732 A-noþer] And
after B   734–35 aftyr … bathynge] *om.* B

and gif here to drynke with white wyne. Or take saffron, galbanum and estorax, of ech a-lich mech half an vnce; stampe hem to-gedir and make of hem as it were a pissary and vse it so.

710

And if the matrice be so hardyd that it holde the floures þat thei may not passe, take lyne-seed and senygrene, of ech an vnce, and tempir it with hony and make a pissary and vse it. To make the floures to come all to the matrice, though the matrice be oute of
715 the right place, and to make hire to conceyue, tak of buttir v ʒ, and juce of jsop ʒ, of [f. 24v] mirre ʒ, of suet of the deer ij ʒ, of grece of an henne ij ʒ, of terpentyne an vnce, and of hony that suffisith, make all these sethe in an 'newe' erthen pott. And vse them vndernethe as a pissary. Ffor this pissary vsed Dame Ffabyan
720 Prycelle whan hire nature was ny wastyd, and she was hool.

And yif ye gyf here ony medicynes, let hire vj or vij dayes a-fore vse metis and drynkys [laxataffis]. And take castorium and temper it with the juce of pulial and of calamynte and gyf hire to drynke, or puliall riall and calamynte and sethe hem in mede and
725 than drye hem and make of hem powder and gif hire to drynke with mede. Dame Cleopatre taught this medicyne to hir dowhter, yif here matrice were so endured and hard that here floures myght not passe; she bad take the galle of a boole or of a-nother beste, and the powdir of nutre [f. 25] and juce of jsope and medill hem
730 to-gedir and than take tosid wulle and make therof a pissary and rolle ther-in and put it in so.

Another: take rue, mynte, puliall riall, of ech a-lyke, iij croppis of sawge, iij plantis of red cole, iij hedis of lekys, and sethe all to-gedyr in a new pot with wyne and gyf here to drynke aftir hire
735 bathynge. Or take tansy, ffethirfoye, mugworte and frye hem in

708 and] or S   mech] + and C   vnce] + & S   712 senygrene] fenygrek S   714 to²] yff S   though ... matrice] *om.* S   715 to²] *om.* S   and] of S   716 suet ... deer] deere suett S   718 make] sethe S   sethe] *om.* S   720 Prycelle] prynces S   721 hire] + vse laxatyue meattis & drynkis S   722 vse ... laxatiffis] *om.* S   laxatiffis] laxtiffis C   724 in] with S   726 with mede] *om.* S   727 here¹] ye S   729 nutre] myrr S   and²] + the S   731 so] *om.* S   733 plantis] cropes S   cole] ꝓ as mvch S   735 ffethirfoye] federfewe S

of louache & þe herbe of nepte & seth them to-gythyre in wynne
& ȝif hare to drynk at euyn ʻ&ʼ at morvnne & let kyuere hare
warme þat sche may svete. Or tak tansay, fethyrfoy, mvgwort &
fry hem in bottyre & bynde hem hot to hare navill & so do ofte.
740 A-noþer þat a Jue dede to þe quene of France: he tok gyngere,
levys [of] lorere & savayn & he stampid hem both to-gythere &
put hem in a pott vp-on quyk colys, & made þe quene to syt ouer
þe pot mowth and receyue þe fume þer-of [vp] in-to hare matryce
& let couyre hare well with clothys þat þe fume myȝht not passe.
745 But whan women vse many suche fumigacyons, hit ys nedfull for
here to anoynt hare wyket with-in with oyle roset for ouer-moche
chafynge.

        Nepte, calamynt, myntis, savayne, eschalones, senvay, pepyre
& comyn be good for hare, vsydde to-gedyre or els eche be
750 hem-selfe. Fovlys of þe felde, kyddys or gottys flesch, fysch
[f. 27] of rynnynge water with scalys, all þeys be good for hare to
ete. And yf sche haue no agu ne feuyre, good hit ys for hare to
drynk stronge whyte wynne. Othyre thyngis were good for hare to
vse but þat woll not I wryht lest summe wolde leue all þes
755 medycynys & vse þat to moche.

        For-to mak þe flovrys to come: let fyrst bath hare & a-nonne
aftyre tak myrre j ȝ & xl cornys of pepyre, staphisagyre vij ȝ &
mak of hem povdyre & ȝiff hare to drynk in wynne, for þat schall
help hare a-non. And tak centory evyn as hit grovyth & stampe hit
760 & mak pelettis þer-of & put hit in-to þe movthe of þe matryce. Or
tak castorium ij ȝ & xv pepyre cornys & stamp hem with wynne &
ȝif hare to drynk in þe juce of pulioll. Or ellys tak dry myntys ij ȝ
& mak powdyre & ȝiff here to drynk in wynne. Or tak colrage &
radysch & sethe them both in wynnc & ley hit to here wyket, as
765 hote as sche may suffure, [f. 27v] & do þat oftyn. Or tak þe
myddyll bark of cherytre & stampe hit & wrynge out þe juce & ȝif

740 þe] a B   741 of] BA, or D   he] *om.* BA   stampid] stampe B   both] *om.* B
742 made] make B   743 pot mowth] mowthe of the pot BA   vp] BA, vt D
745 whan] *om.* B   vse] that vsen B   746 here] theem B   wyket] the mowthe of her
wombe B   ouer-moche] muche B   748 myntis] *om.* B   eschalones] porrett BA
senvay] chybollys, mustarde B   749 &] *om.* B   753 Othyre] o B   754 not I] *tr.* B
wryht] telle B   760 þe²] hyr B   762 in] and B   764 here wyket] þe mowthe of hyr
wombe B   766 of] + the B

botyr and bynde hem hot to hir navill and do it often. A-nother
that a Jue taught [the] queen of Fraunce: he took gynger leuys,
leuys of lorell and saveyn and stampid all a litill to-gedir and put
hem in a pot vpon quyk colys and made the qween to sytte ouer
740 the mowthe of the pot to reseyue the fume in-to here matrice and
let couer hire wel that the fume myght not passe. But what woman
that vsith suche fumigacions, [f. 25v] it is nedfull to a-noynte here
priuite with rue or with oyle roset for ouer-meche chafynge.

745

Nepte, calamynte, myntis, saveyn, porret, eschalons, seneveyn,
pepir and comyn are good for here to vse to-gedir or ech be
750 hem-silff. Ffowlis of the feeld, kyddis or gotis flesh, fysh of
rennynge watir with scalis, these are good for here to ete. And yif
she haue non agu nor feuir, good is for hire to drynke stronge
white wyn.

755

For-to make the ffloures to come: lete firste bathe hire and
a-non aftir tak myrre j ʒ and forty cornys of pepir, [stavesakre] vij
ʒ and make of powdir and gyf hire to drynke in wyn and it shal
helpe here a-non, and take centory as it growith and stampe [it]
760 and make pelotis therof & put it in the mouthe of the matrice. Or
take castorium ij ʒ and xv pepir [f. 26] cornys and stampe hem
with white wyn and gif hire to drynke in the juce of puliol. Or take
drye myntis ij ʒ and make powdir and gif hire to drynke in wyn.
Or tak colrage, radyk and sethe them in wyn and ley it to here
765 priuite, as hote as she may suffre, and do that often. Or take medill
bark of cheritre and stampe it and wrynge owte the juce and gif it

---

737 the] S, *om.* C   738 leuys] *om.* S   stampid] stampe S   all a litill] *om.* S
741 let] *om.* S   what] that S   742 it is nedfull] hathe nede S   748 seneveyn] *om.* S
749 ech] + of them S   751 watir] waters S   752 agu] anger S   good is] jt were
good S   drynke] vse S   757 stavesakre] S, stavysaliv C   758 of] *om.* S   759 it²] S,
om. C   761 xv] *om.* S   766 and¹] *om.* S

hare to drynck iij dayes with whyte wynne.

Ypocras sayth þat yf a woman cast blode at hare movth or have
þe emeroydys or þe fy, þat ys þe cause [that] þe flovyre sekyth to
770 have a way & ys stoppyd & so passyth by wronge wayes. And yf
þe flowre sees for þe defaut of blode, þer is no more for-to do but
make þe woman to ete ofte suche mete as sche desyryth, not
contrary to þe maledy but to hyre luste. And yf the flowr sees by-
cause hit ys stoppyd & may no yssev hav, ye schall mak hem hole
775 in þys manere: let hare vse trifera magna euery ny3ht or ellys
theodoricon anacardinum, for þey be profitabill for þat euyll. Or
ellys theodoricon euperiston þat is most propyr & prouyd for þat,
but for cause hit ys byttyre to taste, wrapp hit in a cole lefe þat be
tendyre sodyn & 3if hit hare. And lette [f. 28] hare blode on þe
780 fote as I have sayd before & mak hare a stew on þys maner. Tak
mugwort, savayne, þe lasse centory, rwe, wormwode, savge,
dauck cretyk, ameos, spica celtica, pulioll, parsly, mynt,
sovthyrnwode & calamynt & boyle all þes erbys be evyn quantite
in a pot & let mak to þe pacyent a subfumigacyon þat sche may
785 receyue þer fume þer-of by-nethe at hare wyket.

Or ellys tak wulle & wrap hit in þe juce of mugwort & rewe &
mak þer-of a pessary & vse hit & 3yf hare euery morvn to drynk
þys drynk. Tak aristologe, longe gencyan, bayes of lorere,
reupontyk, of eche ij 3, sticados, sede of persely, sauge, calamynt,
790 horhownde, camedreos, of eche iij 3 & of dauk, fenell & ache, of
eche j 3, and let sethe all þes to-gethyre in white wynne & 3iff
hare to drynk eche day fastynge.

Medycyns for þe delyuerance of þe secvndyn: yf þe chylde be
borvn & þe secundynne a-byde with-in, let mak [f. 28v] ly of cold
795 watyre & of aschys and clense fayre þe lye & put þer-to j 3 of

---

767 to drynck] *om.* BA   whyte] luke B   769 fy] dropsy B   that] B, of D   770 &[1]
… wayes] *om.* B   771 flowre] flowrys B   þe[2]] *om.* B   for-to] to B   772 ofte]
om. B   773 flowr] flowris B   774 hit] þat that B   hem] hir B   776 theodoricon]
theodoroon B   anacardinum] anacardium BA   þey] these BA   777 ellys] *om.* B
theodoricon] theodoroon B   778 for] by B   hit[2]] *om.* B   779–80 þe fote] her fete B
781 wormwode] *om.* B   782 dauck] dance B   celtica] spicam celticam B
783 sovthyrnwode] *om.* B   &[1]] *om.* B   785 hare wyket] the mowthe of hir wombe.
786 mugwort] + arthemesy B   788 longe] longa B   of] + the B   792 eche day]
om. B

here to drynk iij dayes with lewke wyn.

Ipocras seith that yif a woman caste blood at here mouthe or haue the emerawdys [or] the ffy, that is 'þe' cause of the flouris
770 sekith to haue a weye and is stoppyd and passith be wronge weyes. And if the floures lesse for defawte of blood, than make the woman to ete often suche metis as she desirith, not contrary to the maledy but here luste. And if the floures cesse be-cause thei are stoppyd and may non issew haue, [f. 26v] than let hire vse
775 trifera the grete euery nyght or ellis teodoricioun anacardinum, for these ar profitabill for this euell, or ellis teodoricon empiston that is moste propir and provyd for that, but be-cause it is bitter to taste, wrappe it in a cole lef that is tendir sothen and gif it here; and let hire blood on the foot as is seyd a-fore and make hire a
780 stue on this maner: tak mugwort, saveyn, the lesse centory, rue, wormood, savge, dauc [creticus], ameos, [spicam] selticam, puliol, percell, myrte, sowth-thernwoode and calamynte, boyle thes be euyn quantite in a pot and lete make hire a suffumygacion that she may resseyue the ffume therof at hire priuite.
785

Or ellis take wulle and wrappe in the juce of mugwort and artemesye and rue and make therof a pissari and vse it and lete hir euery morn drynke of this drynk. Also tak aristologe, longe gencian, bayes of lorell, rupontijk, of ech ij ʒ, [sticados], seed of
790 percill, sauge, [f. 27] calamynte, horhond, camedrios, of ech an vnc, of dauce, ffenell and ache, of eche j z, sethe all these in white wyn and gyf here to drynke euery day fastynge.

Yif the child be born and the secundyne a-byde stille with-jn, than let 'make' lye of cold watir and of ashes and clense faire the
795 lye and put therto j ʒ of powdir of malues and gif here to drynke

769 or] S, of C   ffy] fire S   of] *om.* S   774 non ... haue] have none Issewe S   than] *om.* S   776 empiston] empistticon S   777 but] *om.* S   778 taste] tak S   779 as] + it S   781 dauc] daucus S   creticus] S, coelicum C   ameos] *om.* S   spicam] spericum C, spicam *correcting* spericam S;   782 myrte] mynt S   783 lete] *om.* S   787 and¹] *om.* S   788 aristologe] astrologye S   longe] *om.* S   789 sticados] S, disticados C   791 vnc] + ʒ C   dauce] + of S   and ache] *om.* S   792 gyf] + it S

poudyre of malows & ȝif hare to drynk. And so let hare cast &
brak. Or ellys ȝif hare þat povdyre with tisan in warme watyre.
And good ys to stw a woman in þat dysesse with oyle of saltfysch
or oyle of senevy, for þat woll mak þe secvndynne to comme, &
800 blode afture. Or ellys sethe lynsed in water & ȝif hare to drynk.
And yf þe blode comme not afture þe secvndyne, lete [do] to hare
svmme of þe medycyns þat be wryttyn for-to mak þe flowrys to
comme. And yf þe matryce of þe woman ake gretly, tak storax &
good encense, of eche j ȝ, & of þe sede of tovncrassys ij ȝ & lay
805 ham vp-on quyk colys & let hare receyve þe fume.

The signes of prefocacyon or precipitacyon of þe matryce ben
þes: costyfnes, retencion of vrynne, dysesse in þe gret bovell þat
ys clepyd [longaon] & in þe bladdyr, gret akynge of hede & of
[f. 29] raynes, non appetyt, neþer to ete ne to drynk, ne naturall to
810 slepe ne to reste & ofte tym be womet castynge up of mete.
Medycyn for precipitacion of þe matryce: tak þe sede of ache &
þe sede of fenygrek & stampe hit & medyll hit with whyte wynne
& ȝif hare to drynk. An-othyr: tak agaricum & aspaltum & þe sede
of plantaynne & þe sede of tovncrasse & let mak poudyre of all
815 þat and ȝif hare to drynk with wynne & with hony claryfyed.

Hit happyth oþer-whille þat þe matrice commyth so low þat hit
goyth out of þe wyket. The synes of þe whyche ys esy to know,
but wherof hit commyth j schall tell yow. Þat commyth of to
muche colde & to muche moysture & tho fallyn to a woman þat
820 vsyth to sytt longe in a bath of cold water or in a-noþer place
moyste & cold, by þe whyche moysture & cold þe synevs of þe
matryce fallyth & goyth out of hys ryȝht place & so fallyth out,
[f. 29v] & oþer-whille hit fallyth so fore ouermoch enforsement in
þe delyucrynge of chyld.

825   Þe cuere þer-of I schall tell yow: ȝe must vse þe contrary
medycyns þat ye ded in-to þe suffocacyon of þe matryce, þat ys,

798 to] þe B   stw] + to B   801 do] B, to D   803 woman] wombe B   804 &¹] *om.* B
808 clepyd] hyght BA   longaon] B, langao A, logaon D   of²] *om.* B   809 neþer …
drynk] to mete ne drynke B   ne naturall] nor naturally B   810 of] *om.* B   mete]
glit B, gledde A   811 for] + þe B   ache] smalache B   817 of … wyket] at þe mowþe
of the wombe B   818 hit] þat B   822 fallyth¹] slaken BA   hys] þe B   825 þe²]
om. B   826 medycyns] *om.* B   in-to] vse to B   of … matryce] *om.* B

and so let hire caste or brake or ellis gif hire that powdir with a
tesan in warme water. And good it is to stue a woman in that
dishese with oyle of saltfysh or with oyle of senevey, for that will
make þe secundyne to come, and blood aftir. And yif blood come
800   not aftir the secundyne, than do to hire summe of the medicynes
that are wreten for-to make the floures to come. And yif the
matrice ake gretly, tak storax and good encens, of ech a-lyke j ʒ,
and of the seed of ton-cressis ij ʒ and ley hem on qwyk colys and
lete here reseyue the fume.
805

[f. 27v] Sygnes of prefocacion or precipitacion of the matrice ar
thes: costifnesse, retencion of vryne, dishese in the gret bowell
callid longaon and in the bladder, gret akyng of the hed and of the
reynes, non apetite to mete nor drynke nor naturall slepe and often
810   tyme be vomet castyng vp glett. Medycines for thes: tak seed of
ache and seed of ssenygrene, stampe hem and medyll hem with
wyn and gif hire to drynke. A-nother: take [agaricum] and
aspaltum and the seed of plaunteyn and the seed of toncresses and
make a powdir of all thes and gif hire to drynke with wyn or with
815   hony clarifyed.
Othirwhile that the matrice comyth so lowe that it [goethe] oute
at hire priuite and that comyth of to meche cold and to meche
moistour, as to a woman that vsith to sitte longe in bath of cold
watir or in a place moyste and cold throwh the which cold the
820   senewes [f. 28] of the matrice slakyn and go owte of here right
place and so fallith owte. And sum-tyme it fallith so fer ouer the
enforcement and peynynge of deliueraunce of child.

825   Medicynes for this: ye muste vse contrary medicynes that ye
vse to suffocacion of the matrice, that is, all wel savird thynges to

796 and ... hire] so that she S   801 the¹] *om.* S   804 fume] + therof S   809 nor¹] & to
S   810 tyme] *om.* S   thes] this S   811 ssenygrene] venecryke S   812 agaricum] S,
agaritum C   814 make a] *om.* S   of] *om.* S   816 that¹] *om.* S   goethe] S, got C
818 as] & S   821 fer] by S   the] gret S

alle well saverynge thyngis to hare nosse & beneth all [euill]
saverynge thyngis, & tak armoniacum & tempyre hit with þe juce
of wormwode & put hit in-to þe wombe of the woman with
830   pynnys. And þan tak j hand-full of cassie & as moche of rwe & as
moche of mvgwort & seth hit in whyte wynne to þe half & ȝif
hare to drynk. And also mak hote [whete] bren & bynde hit hote in
a bagge to hare navyll & to hare whombe. And yf þe matrice falle
oute & þer be hurte, tak wax terebentynne viij ȝ, of talow of a
835   calfe xvj ȝ, of opium and safrvnne vij ȝ, & a good quantyte of
rosyn. Mak hit thus: mak a pessary & put þe matryce in-to hys
place & afture þat vse þe pessary. And all maner of pessarys
[f. 30] þat been bitter or egyre, a man schold couere hem in woll
& wete hem in oyle or in mylk & so vse ham. There fallyth
840   oþer-whille also in þe matrice a fervent hete, þat hit semyth to þe
woman as hote with-yn as hit were full of brynnynge colys. For
þat euyll ye muste tak oyle of þe white of xij eggys, saffvrne,
mylk of a woman; let menge all to-gethyre & [mynyster] hit with
a pessary.
845   For euyll of þe matryce þat duellyth styll in hys place: tak suet
of a dere, gres of a hogge & of a henne, virgyn [wax], botthyre j ȝ
& aftyrwarde tak fenigrek & lynsede & sethe hem to-gythere on
an esy fyere tyll þey been well sodyn & þan vse ham with a
pessary. Thys is a full good thynge for all euyll þat been with-in
850   þe matryce.

Thys be þe synes of þe retencyon of þe matrice. An hard
suellynge rysyth a-boue þe navill, hare wombe, hare hede & harre
[f. 30v] raynes akyn & þer passyth but lytyll vrynne, gret feavrys

827 euill] well D, evll B   to] into B   830 pynnys] a pyn B, a penne A   cassie]
cresse B   831 hit] hem B   to] into B   832 whete] B, wet D   833 to²] *om.* B   And]
om. B   833–34 falle … þer] *om.* B   terebentynne] + of eche B   835 safrvnne]
+ ana B   839 or] of B   ham] + þere B   839–40 There … whille] *om.* B   840 hete]
+ otherwhile B   hit] and B   þe²] a B   841 of] *om.* B   843 menge] medyll B   all]
+ these B   mynyster] B, mynyst D, vsed A   845 of] in B   846 hogge] gose B,
goys A   wax] BA, wak D   ȝ] of eche a dramme B, *om.* A   847 aftyrwarde] after BA
on] ouer B   849 Thys] that B   full] *om.* B   euyll] evyllis B   þat … with-in] in B
852 Thys] These B   synes] tokyns B   þe²] *om.* B   853 &] *om.* B   854 akyn]
akyng B   feavrys] flewys B, flowes A

hire nose and be-nethe all ill sauyrd thynges. And take aromatum
and tempir it with the juce of wormood, put it in-to here wombe
with a penne. And take [ane] handfull of cassye, as meche of rue
830 and as meche of moodir-woort and sethe them in whyght wyn to
the halff and gif her to drynke. Also make hote whete bren and
bynde it hot in a bagge to hir navill and hir wombe. And yif the
matrice falle owte and ther be hurte, than tak wax [terpentine] viij
3, talwh of a calff xvj 3, de apium & the saffre vij 3, a good
835 quantite of rosyn and make of these a pissary and put the matrice
in-to his place and aftir that vse that pissary. And all maner
[f. 28v] pissaries that are bittir or egre shuld be coueryd in wulle
and wet in oyle or mylke and so be vsed. Ther fallith other-while
in the matrice a fervent hete and that comyth to a woman as hot
840 with-jnne as thowh here matrice were full of brennynge colys. For
this euyll take oyle, the white of xij egges, saffron, mylke of a
woman, menge thes to-gedir and put it in with a pissary.

845   Ffor euyll in the matrice that dwellith stille in his place: tak
suet, grece of a goos and of an henne, virgyn wax, buttir,
ffenygrek and lynseed, sethe them to-gedir in watir and drawe that
juce throwh a cloth, than tak oly and thyngis a-fore seid and sethe
them to-gedir on an esy feer till they be wel sothen and than vse
850 hem with a pissary and this is good thynge for euelys with-jnne
the matrice.
    These are the signes of retencion of the matrice: an hard
swellynge rysith a-boue her navill, hir wombe, hire reynes and hir
hed akyn and ther passyth but [f. 29] litill vryn, grete flowes sue

829 ane] S, and C   cassye] + & S   831 Also] And S   833 and ... hurte] *om.* S
terpentine] S, cerentyne C   834 de] *om.* S   3³] + & S   835 and¹] + of this S
of these] *om.* S   836 his] here S   839 woman] + within S   840 with-jnne] *om.* S
841 oyle] + of S   white] whittis S   847 that] the S   850 this is] thes are S   thynge]
thenges S   853 reynes] hede S   854 hed] reynes S   but] *twice* C

855   sewyn þe purgacyon. The medycynys þat ye have for þe
      suffocacyon been curatyff þer-of & do delyuere yow of þat euyll.

         Thes be þe synnes of þe swellynge of þe matryce: þe woman ys
      suollyn & yf ye thryst hit with yowur fyngyre þe suellynge goyth
      & rysythe sore a-gayne and yf ye smythe on the wombe with
860   yowur hand, hit will sond as hit were a tabure & many soore
      prykyngis & þe wynde rynnyth to and fro in hare body. And in
      svme women hit a-bydyth euer lyche moche. And with sume
      women hit commyth & oþer-whyle passyth and þat euyll
      commyth of cold or ellys of an abhors or ellys yf blode þat schold
865   comme oute with þe chyld whan hit ys borvnne a-bydyth in þe
      movth of þe matryce, for þat will mak hit foule to suell. & þerfor
      let euery woman þat trauelyth be welle ware than whan sche hath
      tra[f. 31]velyd, þat þe humors þat ys wrytyn on þe nexte syde
      comme forth clene. And yf þat thynge sew longe, hit were good to
870   vse of epithyme, dyaspermaton or poliarcon. Or ellys to mak a
      pessary [of] rve & nitrun & pulioll & galle of a bolle & vse hit. Or
      ellys tak fyggis with hare graynes, comyn ʒ ij, & of [affronitri] iij
      ʒ, & mak a pessary.

         Be þys synes schall yow know whan a woman ys nygh hare
875   delyuerance: yn þe vij or viij or þe ix month sche schall have a
      gret heuynesse of bordyn in hare body & in þe raynes, with
      stronge hete & akynge in harre back nygh harre hyppys; þe
      matryce drawth hym donward and hath hys movth more large þan
      hit was wont and when hyre tyme commyth ryʒht neygh, þe
880   partyes a-boue wex-yn small & rysyth gret be-neth & ofte sche
      schall haue talent to mak vryn & moysture drawth dovne to hare
      wyket. And yf sche put in hare fyngere at hare [f. 31v] wyket,
      sche schall fynd þer a humore at þe gretnes of an hen egge, þe

855 sewyn] sewyng B   856 þer-of] hereof B, here for A   do] to BA   þat] þe B
857 þe²] *om.* BA   859 rysythe] restyth B   sore] sone BA   860 a] + belle or a B
862–63 And … passyth] And in some women it comyth & otherwhile passeth and in
some women it abideth ever liche moche B   864 an] *om.* B, a A   abhors] abortyfe B,
horsnes A   865 oute] *om.* B,   870 poliarcon] polyarton B   871 of¹] BA, & D
872 comyn] comyng eueriche B   affronitri] affrotitri DA, a fortigry B   875 or¹] þe B
or²] *om.* B   a] *om.* BA   876 heuynesse] besynesse B   þe] hyr B, here B
880 rysyth] right B, rythe A   882 hare wyket] þe mowthe of her wombe B   in …
wyket] hir finger in to hyt B   883 hen] *om.* B

855 the purgacion; the medicynes that ye haue for suffocacion ar
curabill for this dishese.

These ar the signes of swellynge of the matrice: the woman is
swollyn and yif ye thirste it with your fynger the swellyng goth in
and risith sone a-yen and yif ye smyte on the wombe, it soundith
860 lyke a tabour and many prikkyngis rennyth in the wynde to and
fro in hire body. And with sume women it a-bidith a-lich meche
and summe otherwhile it comyth and otherwhile it passith. And
this euill comyth of cold or of an [abhors] or ellis of blood that
shuld come owte with the child and a-bidith with-jn the mouth of
865 the matrice, for that will make it foule for to swelle. And therfore
war euery woman that trauaylith, that whan she hath trauayled,
that þat humour that is wreten heer-aftir come forth clene. And yif
þat thynge sue longe, it were good of epithym, diaspermaton or
ellis poliarton. And ellis [f. 29v] to make a pissari of rue and
870 vitrum, puliol and the galle of a bole and vse it. Or ellis take
fygges with here greynes, comyn ij ʒ and of [affronitri] ij ʒ, and
make a pyssary.

These are the signes to knowe a woman whan she is ny hire
875 deliueraunce. In the vij, the viij or ix monthe she shal haue gret
heuynesse of berthen in hir body and in hire reynys, with stronge
hete and akynge of hir bak ny hire hipes, the matrice drawith
dounward and hath his mowthe more large than it was wonte. And
whan hire tyme comyth right ner, the partys a-boue wax smale and
880 gret benethe and she hath no talent to make vryn. And moystour
drawith down to hire pryuite and yif she put in hire fynger, she
shal fynde ther an humour at [the] gretnesse of an hennys eg, the
which be-gynneth firste litill and aftir grete and bloody and but

856 curabill] good S   dishese] *om.* S   862 and²] + sum S   863 abhors] hors C,
horse S   865 foule] + & S   866 war] be ware S   867 þat] the S   humour]
humors S   wreten] within S   868 sue] tary S   869 And] or S   870 ellis] *om.* S
871 affronitri] affrotiri C, affrotary S   874 a woman whan] when a woman S   she]
om. S   ny] nere S   hire] + tyme of S   882 the¹] *om.* C, of the S

wyche be-gynnyth fyrst lytyll & aftyr hit be-commyth gret &
885 blody & but hit comme forth whan þe chyld ys borvn, hit ys gret
perell of þe woman, for in soth sche schall sonne afture fall to a
gret sekenes, for hit will suelle in hare marys & tvrne to gret
dysesse yf sche be not holpyn.

The sygnes of þe matryce þat ys gret replet of humors: akynge
890 of eyen & grett het in hare hede & akyng, oþer-will swovnynge &
þe preuy membrys gretly akyn. Medycynne þerfor: tak anneys &
stamp hit & medyll hit with þe gres of a gosse & with bothyre &
þan couer hit in wolle or in lynyn cloth þat be clene & put hit in-to
þe matryce by þe wyket in manere of a pessary. Yf suellynge or
895 oþer wyse falle to þe matryce, þes been the synes: þe pappys
suellynge & be-commyn pale & hard & but medycyn be soner do
þer-[f. 32]to, þe matryce brekyth & moysture passyth & so þe
anguysch passyth lytyll & lytyll & þat makyth þat svmme women
may not conceyue. And hit ys hard to groppe a-bouthe þe matryce
900 & þey swowne ofte for þat cause. And þey woll not suffyre hare
hosbonde to haw do with hem be way of deduit drwere. A
medycyn: tak þe juse of yuy & gresse of a gosse & mak a pessary
þer-of as ye ded to þe matryce þat ys ouer-replet of humors, for
þat ys good for all evylls in þe matryce and vyces.

905 The sygnes of akynge of þe matryce whan þe woman ys
delyuerd of chylde: þe matryce turnyth hym vpward & wexith gret
& all þe body hytt paynyth, where-of sche lyeth oþer-whylle as
ded, but þat hare eyen be not turnyd vpwarde ne þat spetyll
passyth not ne hare synwys be not suollyn but lyeth lyck
910 swownynge. Medycyne for þat malady: tho þat have hit so [f. 32v]
longe tyme & ofte & mow not well endewere þe payne, yt were to
ham to blede vndyr þe ancle. And yf þe paync [lesse], tak
kycumbres & bynd vnto hare flank and yf hit falle of custome to

884 be-commyth] comyth B   885 forth] first B   886 in soth] *om.* B   887 sekenes …
gret] *om.* B   889 of²] with B   humors] + is B   890 hare] þe B   893 in²] clene B
þat … clene] *om.* B   894 wyket] mowthe of þe wombe B   895 wyse] vice B
896 suellynge] swelle B   900 swowne] dremyn B   901 hosbonde] husbondis BA
haw do] dele B   be … drwere] *om.* B   902 medycyn] + therfore B   yuy] rue B
903 ded] doo BA   904 and vyces] *om.* BA   907 body] + þat D   paynyth] + all þe
body D   909–10 but … swownynge] *om.* B   911 þe] *om.* B   912 lesse] lest D, lest
longe B   913 vnto] to B

that comyth foorth whan the chyld [f. 30] is born, it is gret perell
885   of the woman, for she shal sone aftir falle to a gret syknesse, for it
will swelle in here matrice and turne hire to gret dishese but she
be holpyn.

The signes of the matrice þat is ouer-repleet with humours:
890   akyng of jen and gret hete in hir hed and a-kith, other-while
[swownynge] and the prevy membris gretly ake. Than take aneys
and stampe hem and medill it [with] gres of a goos and with butter
and þan couere it in wulle or in lynen cloth and put it in-to the
matrice in the maner of a pissary. Yif swellynge or otherwise falle
895   to the matrice, thes be signes: hire pappis swellyn and be comonly
pale and hard and 'but' medicynes be soner do þer to, the matrice
brekith and moystour passith litill and litill and that makith
sumtyme women may not conceyue, and it is hard to grope
a-bowte the matrice and they swonyn often and they may [f. 30v]
900   not suffre naturally with man. Than take the juce of ivy and grece
of a goos and therof make a pissary as ye do to the matrice that is
ouer-replet of humours.

905   The signes of akynge of the matrice: whan the woman is
deliuerid of child, the matrice [turnethe] vpward and [waxethe]
gret and all the body it peyneth so that she lyth otherwhile as ded,
but that hire yes be not turned vpward nor that spatill passith not
nor hire senewes be not swollyn, but lyth lyk swonynge. Thei that
910   haue this euyll longe and often and may not endure the peyne, it
were good to bleede vndir the ankill, and if the peyne laste, take
kycumbres and bynde hem to here flankis. And yif it falle of
custom to hem and ly longe in swone, than put [to] here nose

884 gret] *om.* S   890 hir] the S   a-kith] akynge S   891 swownynge] S, swowynge C
892 with¹] S, *om.* C   894 the] *om.* S   Yif] + the S   895 swellyn] swollen   900 and]
+ the S   902 of] with S   905 akynge] + of akyng C   906 turnethe] S, turne C
waxethe] S, wax C   907 all ... body] *om.* S   peyneth] + the body S   908 but ...
vpward] *om.* S   nor] so S   909 swonynge] swownyngis S   913 to²] S, *om.* C

hem & ley longe in swowne, put to hare nosse stynkynge thyngis,
915 as ys sayde be-fore where he spekyth of medycyn for þe
suffocacyon. And tak stampydde reu & with hony & oyle mak a
plastre of & lay hit to hare wyket & ofte frote hyre body & namly
by-twene hare leggis. Or tak mustard þat be not to stronge and rub
well harre wombe with-all & hit schall do hare gret ease. And yf
920 hare wyket be hurt, mak a pessary of rosys or of þe povdyre of
rosys & fresch grece of a sowe & þe white of a egge, & vse hit &
aftyre hit mak a subfumigacion of sulphure & þe akyng schall
passe a-nonne.

The synes of þe hardnes of þe modyre þat commyth of a
925 ferwent het þat hath be in þe body of þe woman be-fore: hare
wombe [f. 33] ys euer morre gret suollyn as [thowgh] sche were
with schylde & þe fleche growth gret & hard in here wiket, þat yf
sche put in here fyngyre sche schall fynde þe flesche as harde as
hit were þe hand of a laborere. And oþerwhile þe marys ys so gret
930 þat hit be-commyth as hard as a ston & all þe remenavnt of þe
body ys holdyn with a gret hete.

The sygnes of þe hardnes in þe neck of þe marys ys þis: þe
marys ys mochil opyn, full of akynge & of prykynge, & sche may
not suffure a man tuche here be-twex þe deduit with-out gret
935 grewans & þe flesche of here wiket ys be-comme so hard, as I
have seyd be-fore, þat sche may not feell thowgh a man toche here
here. But þat schall ye hele as ye do þe suellyng of þe marys.

The sygnes of þe boblynge of þe marys ben theyes: hardnes
vndyre þe navill, þe whych yf ye thyrst with yowur fyngere yt
940 wule go dovne & reʹyse vp a-gayne, þe skynne [f. 33v] of þe
wombe ys all hard & yf ye thyrst hit hard þe pacient schall suffyre
gret grevans and whan þe hardnes ys fully gonne þe disesse

914 to] vnto B   915 of] therof B   917 hare wyket] the mowthe of her wombe B
frote] frete B   918 þat] + it B   920 hare wyket] þe mowthe of her wombe B
921 hit] þat B   924 modyre] matryce B, marris A   a] *om.* BA   926 gret] grettly BA
thowgh] thowgth D, thow B   927 here wiket] the mowthe of her wombe B
929 marys] matryce B   930 all] *om.* B   931 a] *om.* B   932 þe¹] *om.* BA   marys]
matrice B   933 marys] matrice B   934 tuche] to deale with B   be-twex þe] by the
way of BA   gret] + gre D   935 wiket] wombe B   936 a man] oon BA   937 here]
there B   marys] matryce B   938 boblynge] bolnenyng B, boylynge A   marys]
matryce B

stynkyng thynge, as is seyd be-fore in suffocacion, and take and
915 stampe [f. 31] rue and with hony and oyle make a plaister ther-of
and ley it to hire priuite. And often frete hire body and namely
betwen hire legges. Or take mustard that is not stronge and rubbe
wel hire wombe and it shal do here ese. And yif here priuite be
hurte, make a pissary of roses or of the powdir of roses and fresh
920 grece of a sowe, and the whight of an eg, and vse it and after make
a suffumygacion of sulphur and the akyng shal passe.

The signes of hardnesse of the matrice that comyth of feruent
925 hete that hath be in the body of þe woman be-fore: hire wombe is
euer gretly swollyn as she were with childe, here flesh growith
gret and hard in here priuite, that yif she put in here fynger she
shal fynde the flesh harde, as it were the hand of a laborer, and
other-while the matrice is so gret that [he] waxith [f. 31v] hard as
930 a ston and all the remanentis of the body is holden with gre't' hete.

Signes of hardnesse in the nekke of the matrice, the which mech
open, full of akyng and prikkyng, and she may not suffre a man
'to' towche hire be the naturall deede, but with gret greuaunce.
935 And the flesh of here priuite is so hard, as I seid a-fore, that she
may not fele thowh she towche there. This euyll ye shal hele as ye
do in the swellynge of the matrice.
The signes of bolnyng of the matrice: hardnesse vnder here
nauyll, on the which yif ye threste with your fynger it will go don
940 and rise vp a-geyn. The skyn of the wombe is all hard and yif ye
threste it sore, she shal fele gret grevaunce and whan the
hardnesse is full gon the dishese passith to the reynes and to hir

---

914 thynge] thengis S   920 after] oft S   921 a] *om.* S   suffumygacion] fumygacyon S
927 fynger] fingers S   929 he] S, *om.* C   930 a] *om.* S   933 akyng] akyngis S
prikkyng] prykkyngis S   934 the] *om.* S   greuaunce] payne S   936 towche] be
touched S   937 in] *om.* S

passyth to hare raynyes & to here forow'ed' & gret hevynes ys
felyd a-boue here schare. That schall 'ye' help as ye do þe
945 suellynge of þe marys, but afture anoynt here with oyle cyperyn.

The sygnes of þe bledyng of þe marys: werynes & smalnes of
þe body, pale colowre as ledde, wamelynge of hart with parlous
blode, for þe pacyentys ben bowndyn with gret dyfficulte &
dryed, & oþer-while þat blode commyth nowth of þe marys but
950 passyth by othyre weyes fro here. Þat bledynge commyth of hard
delyuerance of chylde or ellys of an abors or ellys a vayne ys brok
in here. Medycyn for þat sekenes: mak here to lye on an hard
bedde so þat here fet lye hyere þan here hede & wete a sponge in
cold watyre & aftyre in rose levys & put [f. 34] hit in-to here
955 fowrgeȝ & to here reynes & to hare flank oftyn & let here be
bovnde with wympyls or with othyre softe thyngis & a-noynt here
hede with cold oyle & let here soppe a lytyll aysell & tak þe juse
of plantayne & of morell & put hit in a pessary made with wolle.

The sygnes of þe rynnynge of blode of women owt of mesure:
960 pale colowre, leen of body, gret paynne in goynge, þe body
suellynge, þe fote [bollynge], oþer-whyll þe skyn brekyth, all only
on humor passyth; þat euyll commyth of gret surfet of humors.
Whan þat euyll fallyth with-out wonde or grewance ye schall do
þe same medycynys þat ye do to bledynge of marys. But whan hit
965 fallyth with wonde or with akynge, ye schall mak here hole with
joyce of malovs, with ptysanne & emplaustrys, laxatiuys & with
hote metys & good, for with suche thyngis þe wondys schall be
made hole, all-thow hit comme of to gret fervoor, [f. 34v] þat ys
hete. And yf þe wond be ryȝth foule, þat schall ye wete be þe
970 humor þat passyth, for hit woll fowll stynk & be clere. Tho schall
ye hele as ye do hem þat have þe wondys in þc marys, that ys,

943 hare] þe B   forow'ed'] forger B, folwyth A   944 That] whiche B   schall 'ye']
tr. B   945 marys] matrice B   cyperyn] cypyn B   946 marys] matryce is B   951 an]
om. B   abors] abortyfe B, hors A   ellys²] of B   952 in] with in B   Medycyn]
medicynes B   lye] be B   955 fowrgeȝ] forger B   956 with¹] *om.* B   957 hede]
om. B   þe] *om.* B   959 women] *om.* B   961 fote] fete B   bollynge] bolnyng B,
bolyn & A,   962 humor] humours BA   962–63 of … fallyth] *om.* B   963 wonde or
grewance] *tr.* B   964 marys] matryce B   968 to] a B   fervoor] fervent B   þat ys]
om. B   970 passyth] + from hit B   woll] + be B   stynk] stynkkyng B   be] *om.* B
Tho] þat B   971 þe²] her B   marys] matryce B

forgeth, and gret heuynesse is felte a-boue her share. This euyll ye
shal helpe as ye do the swellynge of the matrice, but after
945 a-noynte hir with oyle ciperyn.

[f. 32] The signes of bleedynge of the matrice: werinesse and
smalnesse of the body, pale colour as led, wamelynge of the herte
with perlous blood; she is bounde with gret difficulte and drye,
otherwhile se that blood comyth not of the matrice but passith
950 other weyes fro hire. That bledynge comyth of hard deliueraunce
of child, or of an [abhors], or that a veyne be broken with-inne
hire. Ffor this euyll lete hire lye on an hard bed, so that hire feet ly
hyer than her hed. Than wete a sponge in cold watir and aftir in
rose leuys and put it in at hire fourgez to hire reynes and to hire
955 flanke and ofte let hire be bonden with wymplis or with other
softe thynges; anoynte hir hed with cold oly and lete hir sowpe a
litill eysell and take the juce of plaunteyn and put it in a pissary of
wulle.

The signes of rennynge of blood owt of mesure: she is pale of
960 coloure, lene of body, swollyn and bollyn, otherwhile the skyn
brekith, only on humour passith [f. 32v] and it comyth of gret
humours. Whan that euill fallith with-oute wounde or grevaunce
ye shal do the medycyn that ye do to bolnynge of the matrice. But
whan it fallith with wounde or with akynge, than take þe juce of
965 malwes with tansy and emplastris, laxatiffis and with hote metis
and good, for with suche thynges the wounde shal hele, thow it
come of feruent hete. And yif the wounde be right fowle, that shal
ye weten be the humour that passith, for it will fouly stynke and
be cleer. This shal ye hele as ye do the woundis of the matrice,
970 that is [to saye with] wax, mirre, fresh grece of an hog and medill
hem to-gedir and make a pissary of wulle and vse it.

---

943 forgeth] fourche S   a-boue] abowt S   946 matrice] + is S   949 se] *om.* S   of]
fro S   951 abhors] an hors C, ane horse S   954 fourgez] fourches S   955 wymplis]
swadbondis S   957 in] + with S   959 rennynge] rysinge S   962 that] the S
964 wounde] wowndis S   965 with¹] & S   laxatiffis] laxatiue S   966 for] fede her S
968 weten] knowe S   fouly] *om.* S   970 to ... with] S, for to C   mirre] *om.* S
fresh] soft S   grece] + & freshe S   an] a S

for-to tak wexe, mirre, fresch grece of a hogge & medyll hem
to-gydyre & mak a pessary & vse hit.

The sygnes of þe slaknesse of þe wyket ben thes: surfet of
975   flourys þat commyth ofte in þe month & þe pacient [hateth] þe
deduit of drewry & yf hit be don to hem a-gayn here will, þey
receyue not þe sede of man. And yf þey receyve hit, þey woyde
hit þe fyrst day or þe ijde & yf hit a-byde & conceyve hit schall be
abors, so þat þe chylde þe ijde or þe iiij monyth formyd schall be
980   but hit schall be sclendyre & lytill, the wyche ye schall helpyn &
hele as ye do þe bledyng of þe marys & þe rynnyng of blode, doth
þe same me[f. 35]dycyns in [such] case, for hit commyth of blode.

The sygne of þe palsy of þe marys ys þis: þe mowth of þe
985   marys schall be hard & thyk so þat thow sche toche hit with here
fyngere sche schall not fel hit & sche schall hate þe deduit of
drewery. And yf sche be takyn forth a-gayne here wyll, sche
schall not conceyve & schall have dysese yn goynge; hyre flouyre
schall be withholdyn or ellys hit schall go owte of mesure & not in
990   dew forme. That schall ye hele as ye do þe bledynge of þe marys
whan hit commyth with akynge & wondys.

The sygnes of mysturnynge of þe marys: the nek & þe movth of
þe marys mow be turnyde in iiij partys, for othyre hit ys turnyde
be-fore or be-hynde or vpward or donward. And yf hit be tornyde
995   donward þe woman may redresse hit with here fyngere. And yf hit
be turnyde vpward or be-fore sche [f. 35v] schall have a suellynge
a-bove here scharre & here vryn schall be disturbelyde to passe.
And yf hit be turnyd donward, the gret vrynne schall passe with
gret noysse & gret paynne & namly yf þat thynge lye nygh þe gret
1000   vrine. The redy sygne of mys-turnynge of þe marys ys thys: þe

974 slaknesse] hurtyng B   wyket] mowth of the wombe B   surfet] surfettis B
975 hateth] B, hath D   975–76 þe³ ... drewry] to deale with man B   978 & conceyve]
om. B   979 abors] abortyffe B, all horse A   chylde] + shall B   schall] *om.* B
980 the] *om.* B   981 þe¹] to B   982 such] scuch D   in ... case] *om.* B   984 sygne]
signes B   þe¹] *om.* B   marys] matrice   985 marys] matrice B   986–87 þe ...
drewery] to deale with man B   988 &] + she B   flouyre] flowrys B   990 hele]
helpe B   marys] matrice B   991 wondys] wounde B   992 marys] matryce B
993 marys] matryce B   997 disturbelyde] distrobeled B   998 donward] + inforthe B
999 &¹] + with B   thynge] thys B   1000 marys] matrice B

The signes of slaknesse of the priuite ar thes: surfet of hir
975 floures that comyth often in the monyth and she hat here naturall
lykyng with man. And yif it be do to hire a-yens hir will, thei
resseyue not the seed of man. And yif thei resseyue it the firste
day or the secund [f. 33] day, and yif it abyde and conceyue it shal
be [abhors], so that the child shal þe secunde monyth or the thirde
980 be formyd, but it shal be slendir and litill. This euyll ye shal helyn
and helpe as ye do the bleedynge of the matrice and the rennyng
of blood: do to the same medicynes in such cas, for it comyth of
blood.

The signes of the palasye of the matrice: the mouthe of the
985 matrice shal be hard and thikke, that yif she towche it with here
fynger she shal not fele it and she shal hate to dele naturally with
man & yif she be take to that a-yens hire wyll, she shal not
conceyue. And she shal haue dishese in goeng, here flouris shal be
with-holden or ellis thei shal go owte of mesure and not in due
990 forme. This shal ye hele as ye do the bledynge of the matrice
whanne it comyth with akynge and wonde.

The signes of mysturnyng of the matrice: the nekke and the
mouth of the matrice mow be turned in-to iij parties, [f. 33v] ffor
otherwhile [it] is turned be-fore or be-hynde or vpward or
995 dounward, she may redresse it with hyre fynger. And yif it be
turned dounward, she may redresse it with hyre fynger and yif it
be turned vpward or be-fore, she shal haue a swellynge vpon hir
shar and hire vryn shal be disturbyd to passe. And if it be turned
donward hindforth, the gret vryn shal passe with gret noyse and
1000 peyne and namely if it ly ny the gret vryn. The redy signes of

---

975 hat] hathe S   976 thei] she S   977 resseyue¹] concevithe S   978-80 and¹ ... litill]
om. S   979 abhors] all hors C   980 euyll] *om.* S   ye shal] *tr.* S   981 and helpe]
om. S   981-83 and¹ ... blood] *om.* S   984 the palasye] mysturnynge S   987 naturally
with man] with man naturallye S   993 mow] may S   994 it] S, *om.* C   995 fynger]
fingers S   995-96 And ... fynger] *om.* S   999 hindforth] than S   1000 ny] one S

moysture rynnyth owte of þe marys othyre-while white & watery
& oþer-whylle rede or blody or black; oþer-whylle hit passyth
with gret dysesse, othyre-whylle with no dysesse.

 Medycyn for þat euyll: ȝiff here to drynk papauere with whyte
1005 wyne. Aftyre stamp þe scalys of eggys & mak a pessary. And yf
þe marys be mevydde owte of hys plasse, tak wex & sevet of a
deere evyn mesure, vij ȝ of terebentynne, of gresse of a gosse
euyn lyck iiij ȝ, & a lytyll of [opyon] & tempyr all to-gethyre with
oyle cyperyn & vse hit in a pessary, for þat pessary ys helpynge to
1010 a maledy þat is clepyd þe fyere of helle, þat rysyth of colere &
all-so to oþer apostemys & prykkyngis & hurtys with-in þe marys
& to many othyre thyngis all-so.

 And be-cause þer be many maner of apostemys, both on a man
& woman, I will wryt to yow in what maner ye schall know on fro
1015 a-noþer. For ryȝth as þer be diuerse humorys in þe body of man,
so þer be diuerse apostemys þat be callyd in Englysch boches or
bleynes. Oon commyth of blode & hit is callyde flegmon in
Frenche. An-oþer commyth of colere & ys callydde herpes
omenus. The iij commyth of melancholy & ys calde cancer. The
1020 iiij commyth of flewme & ys callyd zimia. And þes apostemys
schall ye know be thes sygnes: yf þe apostem come of blode, hit
schall be rede & þe pacient schall have a gret het. And yf þe
apostem comme of flewm, hit schall be whyte & softe & yf ye
presse yowur fyngere þer-on, þe hole þat ye mak will not sone
1025 rysse. And yf þat apostem be of rede [f. 36v] colere, hit schulde be
of citryn colore. And yf hit comme of melancoly or of black
colere, þe apostem will be black & hard. And yf hit comme of
blode, hit ys good to blede in hast. And yf hit comme of oþer wey,
purge hem by medycynys laxatiuis.

1001 marys] matrice B 1002 rede] wete B or[1]] and B 1003 othyre-whylle …
dysesse] *om.* B 1004 to] *om.* B papauere] purpure B 1005 scalys] shalys B
1007 of[2]] and BA 1008 opyon] opyn D, opium BA 1009 hit] that B to] of B
1010 helle] + that is apostem B rysyth] aryseth B of[2]] to B 1011 apostemys]
postemys B &[1] … hurtys] that prikkys B marys] matryce B 1013 apostemys]
postemys B 1017 bleynes] bylcs BA hit] þat B 1018 An-oþer] + and he B
1018–19 herpes omenus] herbesyti B, jmpensethy onnenus A 1020 callyd] + zimna
or B apostemys] + my ladye A 1022 a] *om.* B 1024 þat] *om.* B 1028 ys good]
tr. B of] by BA

mysturnynge of the matrice ar thes: moystoure rennyth owte of the matrice othir white and watry, other-while red and bloody, otherwhile it passith with gret dishese.

Than gif here drynke papauery with white wyn and after stampe
1005 the shalis of eggis with wyn and make a pissary. And yif the matrice be mevyd owt of þe place, than take wax, suet of a deer euyn mesure, vij ʒ of terpentyne, grece of a goos euyn lyke iiij ʒ, a litill of apium and tempir all to-gedir with oyle ciperyn and vse in a pissary, ffor that [f. 34] pissary is helpynge to any maladye that
1010 is callid fier of helle, that is a-postem that risith of [colour] and also to other ʼaʼpostemys, as prykkynges and hurtyngis and hurtis with-in the matrice and to many other thynges.

[And] be-cause þer are many maner of apostemys, both on man and woman, heer may ye knowe how ye shal knowe on fro
1015 a-nother. Ffor right as ther be diuers humours with-jnne the body of man, so be ther diuers apostemys that are callyd in the Inglish bocchis or belys. On comyth of blood and that is callid fflegmon in Frensh. Another comyth of [colore] and that is callid herpesethi omenus. The thirde comyth of malecoly and is callid the cankyr.
1020 The fourte comyth of flewme and that is callid zimia. And thes apostemys shal ye knowe be signes heer folwynge. Yif aposteme come of blood, it shal be red and þe pacient shal haue gret hete. [f. 34v] And if the aposteme come of flewme, it shal be white and softe and yif ye presse your fynger ther-on, the hole that ye make
1025 wil not sone rise. And yif the posteme be [of] red colour, yt shuld be of citryne colour. And yif it come of malecoly, the aposteme will be blak and hard, and if it come of blood, good it is to bleede in haste. And yif it come be other weyes, purge hym with medicynes laxatiffis.

1004 here] + to S   1005 make] vse it as S   1008 in] it as S   1009 any] a S
1010 callid] + the S   colour] S, colry C   1011 ʼaʼpostemys] postumes S   hurtis]
hurtyngis S   1013 And] S, nd C   maner of] *om.* S   on] of S   1014 ye shal] to S
1015 Ffor] And S   1016 the] *om.* S   1017 belys] byles S   1017-18 blood ...
Another] *om.* S   colore] S, colry C   that] *om.* S   1019 omenus] + one comethe of
bloud & that is called flegmon in frenche S   1020 that] *om.* S   1021 heer] *om.* S
aposteme] the apostem S   1024 presse] put S   ther-on] that C   1025 be of] be C,
come of S   shuld] shal S   1026 of'] *om.* S   1027 good ... is] it is good S
1028 come] rvn S   hym] hem S   with] + hym with C   1029 medicynes laxatiffis]
mediycyne laxatyue that ar for the humours S

1030   To apostem þat commyth of blode, mak þys emplaustre. Tak
comyn bresyde, gresse of beere, wete-mel, rew, oynons sodyn,
mengyll thys thyngis sodyn in wyn & in oyle longe till þey be
made thyk & aftyre bynde them on þe apostem as a emplaustre till
hit be well rypyd & softe & þan lawnce hit at þe most hongynge
1035 place, þan put a tent þer-in of feyre lynett & ley þer-to salvys as
ye do to oþer wondys. The apostemys or an antrax or a carbunkyll
þow schall hell with colde thyngis, as ys oyle roset, joyse of
morell & þe celydon whyld.

    Thys thyngis schall þow put to a empostem but yf hit comme of
1040 blode: ley þer-to scabios, for that ys a provyd thynge for þat & þe
[f. 37] lytyll daysey meddyld with dovys donge ys good. And yf
þe apostem be of red colere & be hot & dry & yf hit be in a place
& ʿþat hitʾ mak a gret wond, þow schall mak hit hole as thow do
an antrax. And yf þe apostem come of flevme, mak þis
1045 emplaustre. Tak ix rotys of white malow & sethen them well with
viij ʒ of gresse olde of pork & ij quantite of oyle & when þe rotys
be well sodyn, þan draw þe lyqure thorow a cloth & put þer-to ix ʒ
of litarge & let seth hit on colys & stere hit well & aftyre ley hit to
þe apostem in maner of a emplaustre.

1050   Or ellys mak a emplaustre on þis wyse, for hit will [rype] all
apostemys. Tak þe brawnchys of branck vrsyn & þe rotis of white
malow & sethe þem well in water & aftyre stamp hem well with
olde gres of a pork & put þat to buttyre, wynne, mylk of a woman,
& mak þer-of a emplaustre. Or ellys take þe white with þe ʒolk of
1055 a egge & salt & mak a emplaustre. Or ellys tak lyly rotis [f. 37v]
& sethe þem in water & stamp hem with olde gres of a hogge &
oynyns sodyn, with whylde celydony & þe levys of colys &

1031 bresyde] brosed B, brossed A   wete-mel ... onyons] whete medled in hony
onyon B   1032 mengyll] medyll BA   1033 on] vnto B   emplaustre] plaister B
1034 þan] + lett B   1035 place] *om.* B   1036 The] These BA   1037 with] + a B
thyngis] thyng B   1038 & ... whyld] wylde celydonye B   1039 schall þow] *tr.* B
empostem] aposteme B   1042 be¹] come B   1043 &] *om.* B   thow] ye B   1044 þe]
om. B   1045 emplaustre] plaister B   white] wylde B   malow] malowes B
1046 gresse olde] *tr.* B   pork] a porker B   quantite] quartis B   1046–47 &² ... well]
om. B   1047 þe] *om.* B   1049 emplaustre] playster B   1050 emplaustre] playster B
on] in B   wyse] maner B   rype] B, *om.* D   1051 white] wyld B   1052 with] in B
1053 olde] *om.* B   þat] þer B   buttyre] + & B   wynne] + & B   1054 ʒolk] yelow B
1055 emplaustre] plaister B   ellys] *om.* B   1056 hogge] porke B

1030   For aposteme that comyth of blood mak this enplastire: take comyn brosid, grece of a bor, whete-mele, rue, onyons sothen, medill thes to-gedir in wyn and oly longe till thei be thikke and aftir bynde them to the apostem as a plastir till it be wel ripe and softe; than let it be launcyd at the moste hengyng place and than
1035 put a tent ther-in of fair lynt and ley ther-to salues as ye do to other woundys. [f. 35] These apostemys, antrax or carbuncle, ye shal hele with cold thyng, as is oyle roset, juce of morell, celidony welde.

     And yif it come of blood, ley ther-to scabious, for that is prouyd
1040 thynge for þat, and the litill dayesje medelid with dowes donge is good. And yif the aposteme come of red colour and be hot and drye and yif it be in place that it make a gret wounde, than shal ye hele it as ye do an antrax. And yif the aposteme come of flewme than make this plaistir. Take ix rotis of wyldemalwe and seth hem
1045 wel with viij vnce of olde grece of an hog, ij quantite of oyle and whan the rotis be wel sothen, than drawe the licour throw a cloth and aftir put therto ix vncis of lytargion and set it on colys and stere it well and aftir ley it to the aposteme in maner of a plaister.

1050 Or ellis make a plaister on this maner, for it will rype all empostemys. [f. 35v] Tak the braunchis of vrsyn, the rootis of [wyldemalwe] and sethe them wel in watir and after that stampe hem in olde grece of an hog and put ther-to buttir, wyn and mylke of a woman and make therof a plaister. Or take the white with the
1055 yello of an eg and salte and make a plaister. Or take lyly rootis and [put] them in watir and stampe hem with grece of an hog and onyons, with wylde selidonye and the leuys of colys and lynseed

1030 For] + ane S   1031 grece ... bor] bores grece S   1032 oly] boyle them S 1034 be] + well S   hengyng] rypest S   1035 to] + the S   1036 antrax] *om.* S carbuncle] carbocles S   1037 thyng] thengis   is] *om.* S   celidony] + and C 1038 welde] *om.* S   1040 thynge] *om.* S   1043 an] a carbocle or S   1044 ix] the S 1045 vnce] vnces S   olde] *om.* S   ij] twyse the S, + *lacuna* C   1047 therto] + an C 1048 stere] store S   1051 vrsyn] vyne & S   1052 wyldemalwe] wylmalwe C, wild malows S   1053 grece ... hog] hogis grece S   1055 yello] yolke S   lyly] lely S 1056 put] S, *om.* C   in] into S   grece ... hog] hogis grece S   1057 selidonye] celydon S

lynsede sodyn with whynne: all þes thyngis been good to ryppe apostem, eche by hymselfe or ellys all to-gethyre.

1060   And summe-tyme hit fallyth þat cancvrs fallvn to women as þey do to men. And þerfore I schall tell yow how they comme. Othyrwhille þey comme of humors þat been rotydde with-inforth & othyre-whille þey [fallyn] outward of wondys or of sorys þat be not well helyd. For a wonde þat semyth helyd iiij dayes or v, &
1065   brekyth ovte a-gayne, schulde not be callydde a wonde but a kankyre or a fystere. And oþer-while hit fallyth þat a cankere [is] new & othyrwille olde & othyre-whille in a playnne place full of flesch & oþer-whille a-monge synneve, & þan a man schall do curys to hem by no cuttynge ne by no fyere.

1070   Tak schepys dong & poudyre of comyn & franckensensse & mak of [f. 38] all þes poudere; þan tak a tille & hete hit & cast þer-on of þe poudere & stev þe on & vse þis on moroue & on eue. And for-to a-wayle þe maris smell to asafetida & þis medicyn is preuydde.

1075

    A fayre medycyn for a woman þat hath to moche of here floures, to lesse hem. Tak comfire and wasch hit, stamp hit & sethe hit in wynne & mak a emplaustre þer-of & ley hit to here navyll & to here wombe & to here raynes & sche schall be hole.

1080   For-to mak a woman to have here floures, but look sche be not with childe. Tak þe rot of gladyn & sethe hit in vynegyre or in wynne & whan hit is well sodyn, set hit on þe grovnde & let here stride þer-ovyre so þat þer may no aiere a-waye but in-to here priuite.

1085   A medycyn for a woman þat hath to moche of here floures. Tak plantayne, bursa pastoris, letuse, of eche lyck moche, & boyle hem in fayere water & with that water tempure blavnchide almondes [f. 38v] & mak mylk & whan ye will ete þer-of; boyle

1059 eche] *om.* B   1060 þey] hit B   1063 fallyn] favllyn D, fallen B   1063–64 or … a] *om.* B   1066 is] B, *om.* D   1067 othyrwille] other B   a] *om.* B   1068 synneve] synewes BA   1069 curys] cure B   to] *om.* B   1070 Tak … *end*] *desunt* A   &²] *om.* B   1071 a] + litell B   1072 on¹] ther over B   moroue … on³] *om.* B   eue] evenys B   1073 maris] matrice B   1077 hit¹] *om.* B   hit²] + clene B   1078 emplaustre] plaister B   1083 stride] stonde B   1086 &] *om.* B   1088 &²] *om.* B ye] she B

sothen with wyn: all these thynges ar good to ripe aposteme be [þem]-selff or ellis all to-gedir.

1060   And sumtyme it fallith to women as wel as to men. And tho otherwhile come of humoures that arn rotyn with-jnne forth and other-while they falle owtward as woundis or sorys that be not wel helyd iiij dayis or v, and breke owte a-yen, shal not be callid a wounde but a kankyr or a festre. And otherwhile it fallith that a

1065 kankyr is newe and otherwhile olde and [f. 36] otherwhile pleyn place ful of flesh and othirwhile a-monge senewes, and than a man shal do cure hem be no cuttynge nor be no fire.

1070   A medycine prouyd for the white floures of wyf or maydyn, to stoppe hem yif they come to surfetously. Take oyle benedictum ȝ ij, oyle of lyly ȝ j, oyle of camamyll ȝ j, medyll thes to-gedir and aftir the rede be gon a-noynte here syde wher she felith moste peyne, and the reynes of hire bak, and a litill on hir navill, and wel

1075 on hir body a litill a-boue hire share.

   Explicit

1058 ripe] + an S   1059 þem] them S, þe C   all] *om.* S   1060 women] a woman S wel as] *om.* S   tho] *om.* S   1061 otherwhile] + it S   1062 or] & S   1064 that] to S 1065 is] as S   pleyn] *twice* C, in a S   1067 do] + no S   hem] *om.* S   no[1]] *om.* S 1070 or] + of S   maydyn] mayd S   1071 to] *om.* S   oyle] oleum S   1077 Explicit] *om.* S

hit a lytyll & put sugyre þer-in & whan ye will ete ryse potage, ye
1090 may tempire hit with þe mylke forsayde.

A bath for þe same sekenes: tak welewyn levys, goldys clot
leuys, rose leuys, louach, malovs & plantayne, sethe þis herb in
water, þan bath yow in þat water so þat hit be not to warme. And
when ye hawe be þer-in as longe as ye luste, than tak water þat is
1095 sumwhat coldyrre & wasch clene all yowur body þer-with. And ye
may vse in somer as longe as ye lyst; but suet not in yowur bath.

Dyetynge for the same evyll: ye may ete hen, capon, fesawnt,
perterych & all maner whilde foule of þe feldys & wodys, saue
hole fote foulys. And ye may ete well moton, kydde, lambe, pork
1100 of j yere olde & rabbettis, & ye may ete pochydde eggys & ye
may ete þe brovesse of capon broth & jussell & tooys of a capon
[f. 39] and collys of oþer fovlle fore-nemydde, and stvys & brothis
made of þe fleschis forsayde. And ye may ete all maner of fysch
of fresch water, saue elys & tenchys.

1105 Tak mirre, gentian, bayes, aristologe longe, of eche ijd & þan
mak them in povdyre & þan put to that poudere of þe syruppe of
wormwode as moche as sufficith to mak a balle & gyf þer-of at
onys to þe pacient jd worth or morre. Thys is to putte out þe
secundine or aftyre-byrth.

1089 ye¹] she B   1090 þe] *om.* B   forsayde] aforesaid B   1091 welewyn] wyld
vyne B   1092 þis] these B   herb] herbys B   1093 water¹] + & B   1096 vse] + þis
bathe B   1098 perterych] pautryke B   maner] + of B   &²] + of B   1099 fote]
fotyd B   1100 &² ... ete] *om.* B   1100–01 &³ ... þe] *om.* B   brovesse] brewes B
tooys] colys B   1102 of] + eny B   fore-nemydde] afore-nemyd B   1103 forsayde]
afore-said B   1103–04 fysch ... water] fresshe watyr fysshe B   1105 ijd] ij peny
worthe B   1106 of⁴] *om.* B   1107 gyf] *om.* B   1108 onys] + gyffe B

Commentary

Line numbers, lemmata, and comments refer to the Douce text and by implication to the corresponding passage in the Cambridge text, unless otherwise stated. All quotations from the Old French translation of *LSM* 1 are from the version in BL MS Sloane 3525, and are referenced by folio number and column. All quotations from the Muscio derivative *Non omnes quidem* (M) are taken from Oxford Bodley MS Laud Misc. 567, fols 62r–66v, and are referenced by the chapter numbers based on the index on fol. 62r (see above, pp. 21–22). References to the *Genicia Cleopatrae* (C) are also from the version in MS Laud Misc. 567, fols 58v–60v, and are by folio number.

1–9 *Ovre ...iiij:* 'Quant deus nostre seignor out le mund estore, sor tote creature si fist home raisnable .... Si commanda a creistre et a multeplier et establi ke des deus uendreit le tierz, et del cors del home, qui plus est de chaude nature et de seche, istrent la semence en la feme, [et la feme] ke plus est de freide nature et de mole la recoeureit et par la temprement del chalt et del freit et del sec et del moiste creistrent li enfes. Ices quatre choses sunt necessaire as herbes et as arbres et as blez.' (fol. 246vb) The ME is clearly following Fr. rather than the Latin text *LSM* 1, which is longer and more complex here (see Hunt, *Anglo-Norman Medicine*, p. 116, and *The 'Trotula'*, ed. Green, 'Liber de Sinthomatibus Mulierum' [1]).

9–12 *And ... gendrynge:* 'Mais pour ce ke les femes sunt de plus fieble qualite ke li ome et ount greignor trauail d'enfant, pour ce lor auienent plusors enfermetez ke as homes, et maiesmement a cels membres ki a l'engendreure apertienent.' (fol. 246vb)

13 *Wherfore ... sayntys:* Note that these pious sentiments are an addition of the ME redactor and are not in Fr.

13–18 *I ... Latyn:* 'Et pour ce ke femes sunt plus huntoses de dire lor enfermetez as homes ke as femes, si lor faz icest liure en language ke eles l'entendent, que les unes sachent les altres aidier. Bien sachent que ie i met del mielz ke lor besoigne a lor enfermetez que ie ai trouue des diz Ypocras et Galien et Constentin et Cleopatras et ici troueront dont li mal / uienent et comant porront guarir.' (fols 246vb–247ra) Again, the Fr., which is closely followed by the ME, has considerably adapted *LSM* 1 (Hunt, *Anglo-Norman Medecine*, p. 116, cf. *The 'Trotula'*, ed. Green, 'Liber de Sinthomatibus Mulierum [2]). It is interesting that the ME redactor abbreviates the conventional topos of 'women's shame' (that they are embarrassed to expose their maladies to male physicians) and instead places much more emphasis on women's linguistic disadvantages: that they are either illiterate or, if literate, can read only the vernacular. The ME is also far less specific (or boastful) about the details of his sources.

24–31 *And ... hevyn:* Not in Fr. Again, the addition is conventionally pious but slightly sinister at the same time.

32–37 *[R]yht ... conceyue:* Cf. 'si li a Nature establi un espurgement ke l'on apele flos pour ce k'ele ne puet conceuoir sanz ice plus que li arbres fruit porter se einz ne florist.' (fol. 247ra)

þe makere of all þyngys: Fr. 'Nature'; another example of the orthodox religious tendencies of the ME.

34 *esporgymente*, C *espurgement:* Adopted unmodified from the Fr. *espurgement*. MED does not list *espurgement*; it does have the normal ME reflex, *purgement*, but gives only a spiritual, not a medical or scientific, meaning.

37–39 *For ... woman:* 'Icest espurgement auient a la feme altre si com al home auient pollucion pour habundance des humors.' (fol. 247ra)

39 *as ... here-aftyre:* That is, at 187 seq.

40–51 *But ... maryce:* This passage on the differences between men and women is not in Fr.; its purely empirical nature suggests it may be the ME redactor's own contribution (see General Introduction, p. 8).

60–77 *hit ... cuntreys:* The theory of the seven-chambered uterus was widespread in the Middle Ages, 'found in Latin anatomical and embryological texts as early as the twelfth century. It is not found in gynecological texts, however, until the late Middle Ages' (Green, 'Obstetrical and Gynecological Texts', p. 85 n. 76). It appears in *The Nature of Wommen*, a ME version of an abbreviated translation of Muscio misleadingly entitled *Trotula de naturis mulierum*: 'Þer ben .vij. resseyuyngys of nature with inne þe matryce, þat is to say .3. on þe on syde and .3. on þe oþir syde, and .on. in þe myddys with inne al þe oþir .vj' (Green, 'Obstetrical and Gynecological Texts', p. 85). It is also found in the Middle English translation of the pseudo-Galenic *De Spermate:*

> It is to be noted that a womman hath vij cellis or receptacles where sperme is received. ... if sperme fal in the right side of the matrice, it shal be a man .... If sperme falle in the lift side, it shal turne into femynyne nature ....

(*Medieval Embryology in the Vernacular: The Case of 'De Spermate'*, ed. by Päivi Pahta, Mémoires de la Société Néophilologique de Helsinki 53 (Helsinki: Société Néophilologique, 1998), p. 173).

67–69 *And ... conceyvydde:* Not in Fr. or *Non omnes quidem.*

88 *precipitacion*, C *precipitation:* The meaning 'prolapse', which seems appropriate here, is not in MED or OED, which give no medical senses.

prefocacion: Glossed by MED as 'suffocation' or 'strangling', the meaning given by Lewis & Short for Lat. *praefocatio*. However the ME word seems to have a different meaning from *suffocacyon* that is closer to *precipitacion*. Context suggests that it means 'sideways displacement', as opposed to both displacement upwards (suffocation) and displacement downwards (precipitation).

103–04 *svmme ... dayes:* 'Non omnes quidem equaliter purgantur, sed quedam plurimis, quedam paucis diebus.' (M1)

107 *fro ... yere*, C104–05 *This ... age:* See D. W. Amundsen and C. J. Diers, 'The Age of Menarche in Medieval Europe', *Human Biology*, 45 (1973), 363–69, where the various ages given in medieval texts are summarized. They note that manuscripts of Trotula texts give the age variously as 13, 14, and even 15 (as here) and conclude: 'the age at menarche during medieval times approximated that of the classical period and that currently reported in

Europe. Except for the infrequent reports of the fifteenth year of life as an upper limit, there is no evidence that the retardation of age at menarche, evidenced at the end of the 18th century, had yet begun' (p. 368).

107–08 *till ... olde:* See D. W. Amundsen and C. J. Diers, 'The Age of Menopause in Medieval Europe', *Human Biology*, 45 (1973), 605–12. They note the wide variation in age at menopause found in medieval texts: ages between 35 and 75 can be given but 50 is most frequently cited. They comment: 'The observations on age at menopause made by medieval sources ought not to be labeled as absurdities. ... many medieval sources evidenced a very healthy independence of thought that probably resulted in their openness to observation even when it led to the discarding of venerated authority and tradition' (pp. 610–11).

113–129 *Now ... passe:* The outline of this section is to be found in *Non omnes quidem* (M1). The list of classes of women who do not menstruate is slightly rearranged, and considerably expanded in detail.

114–16 *Women ... flovrys:* 'Que uero in utero habent, ex ipso sanguine infantem nutriunt.' (M1)

116–17 *tho ... blode:* 'Que autem egritudine afficiunt, sanguine simul cum uirtute priuantur.' (M1)

117–18 *Ne ... moche:* Mistranslation of 'uel que ... laborant'.

119–21 *tho ... wastyth:* A conflation of 'que in choro cantant' and 'Que uoce exercentur, sanguis earum ex ipsa exercitatione consumitur.' (M1) For the idea that this applies to religious women (who of course 'sing in choir'), compare *The Nature of Wommen*, 'Wommen of relegion purge noght because of rysyng o nyght and synggyng and ocupacyon in her seruyse her blod wastyth' (Green, 'Obstetrical and Gynecological Texts', p. 86). Green comments that, along with the reference to the seven-chambered uterus (see note to 60–77) this idea that 'religious women, more than others, have a propensity toward amenorrhea' is the only major element in *The Nature of Wommen* not found in its Latin source (p. 85). See further Green p. 86 n. 78, and Barratt, 'Translation and Censorship', pp. 317–18.

123 *Ne maydyns:* 'Puelle uero'. (M1)

127–28 *women ... age:* 'et anus'. (M1)

135–38 *But ... chylde:* Most versions of the Latin Trotula do include contraceptive recipes: see P. P. A. Biller, 'Birth-Control in the West in the

Thirteenth and Early Fourteenth Centuries', *Past & Present*, 94 (1982), 3–26, and Monica H. Green, 'The Development of the *Trotula*', p. 131.

139–53 *suffocacyon ... dede:* The subject is dealt with further at D530–82.

154–71 *Precipitacion ... slepe:* These observations are developed further at 816–24, but quite different causes are given there for the condition, suggesting that the ME is using two separate sources.

C200 *menstrualis:* D has Anglicized this word but C has kept the Latin form (though there is no known Latin source at this point).

208–13 *And ... vaynes:* Cf. 'l'en uient a la fiee pour ce ke la marriz est desnaturee et refroidiee, et a la fiee de ce ke les ueines de la marriz sunt grailes, com ount les graisles femes, et ke les humors n'ont ueie par quoi eles puissent passer, et a la fiee de ce que les humors sunt espesses et engluees et ne pueent eissir.' (fol. 247rb)

215–17 *And ... be-nethe:* Cf. 'a la fiee de ce que li sanc ist del cors par altre liu, com de cele ki a le fi ou di cele que li nes siegne souuent ou de cele ki le sanc escopist.' (fol. 247rb) There is no mention of haemorrhoids (*emeroydys*) in Fr. but they are mentioned in *LSM* 1 (Hunt, *Anglo-Norman Medecine*, p. 117, 'per ficus sive emoroydas', *The 'Trotula'*, ed. Green, 'Liber de Sinthomatibus Mulierum' [7]). This suggests that MS Sloane 3525 was not the copy of the Fr. text actually used by the ME translator.

223–35 *Now ... pale:* Cf. 'Ce ke la feme a trop de ses flors .... Ice auient a la fiee de ce ke les ueines de la marriz sunt ouertes. A la fiee crieuent les ueines et ce est quant li sanc est ha/stiuement roges et clers; et a la fiee de ce ke la feme a coilli trop sanc de trop mangier et de bouire et de trop grant repos .... A la fiee de ce ke li sanc est trop eschaufez por les coles qui issent del fiel, si se meslent od le sanc, s'il eschaufent, s'il funt boillir, si ke les ueines nel pueent tenir ne soffrir. Se ce ki ist de la naisance est de coles, donc torne il a ialnor; se ce est de flieme, si est de blanche color; se ce est de sanc, si est rouge.' (fols 248va-b)

236–44 *An-oþer ... in-curabyll:* Cf. 'Ice mal auient quant li sanc de tot le cors est corrumpuz, si nel puet retenir por sa maluestie, et por ce ke il est desnature. A la fiee auient icest mal d'auotier et de ce muerent femes souuent. Quant icest mal soprent feme, ele pert la color et le mangier et en amaigrist; se longuement li dure, si li torne a ydropisie por ce ke le foi en refreidist por le sanc ke il pert.' (fol. 248vb) ME omits the reference to abortion as one cause of this condition and of maternal mortality.

249–53 *Now ... kynde:* 'Quandiu puelle uirgines esse debeant. Donec purgatione superueniente, natura possit et matrix officia sua adinplere.' (M2) A sudden change of subject, and of source, from the Fr. version of *LSM* 1 to *Non omnes quidem* derived from Muscio. The English texts have already (D123–24) specified 15 as the age of menarche.

250 *dewery:* MED gives no forms without -r- for *drewery*, but the appearance of this spelling twice (again at D484) suggests that it is not an error but formed by dissimilation.

256 *lauy:* Probably a form of the uncommon word *lavei* (possibly derived from Celtic). MED glosses it as '?Noisy ?unruly'; the illustrative quotation suggests it means 'boisterous' or 'uncontrollable'.

259–64 *Now ... mery:* 'Que sint apte ad concipiendum. Hec scilicet que <in>ordinabiliter die suo purgantur limpido et moderato sanguine et que orificium matricis rectum et proximiorem habent; corpusque omne neque nimis durum neque ualde digestum, cum integritate anime et hilaritate.' (M3)

264–66 *go ... conceyve:* '[Quid] [MS Quod] tempus sit aptius ad concipiendum. In declinatione scilicet purgationis, dum subiaceat coitus desiderio et ita ut neque habundantia cibi plenum habeat corpus ... et si sic post curationem corporis misceatur, saluberrima erit conceptio.' (M4)

267–71 *Now ... wrath:* There is nothing in *Non omnes quidem* that corresponds to this section on the care of the pregnant woman before the last trimester. This seems to be the translator's own addition although some of the material is similar to that found in *The Nature of Wommen:*

> And .vij. monethes lat hyr noght go to faste ne trauayle to sore on no maner werk for mys pressyng and contreynyng of hyr body for doute of castyng out of þe norechyng of þe schyld, þe wheche wyl falle out with constreynyng.

(Green, 'Obstetrical and Gynecological Texts', p. 87). The addition throws light on the intended readers of the ME version. They were clearly women of the leisured class, able to enjoy the luxury of not engaging in physical work during pregnancy, and who had access to horses and might normally expect to ride (fast, apparently). The translator also evinces a very 'modern' belief in the influence of negative emotions on the physical health of pregnant women.

268 *restely,* C *restly:* The meaning is clear enough from the context but MED does not record the word. OED records it, but with the sense 'stubbornly', from 1611.

272–73 *& ... passe:* 'Quomodo vii mense agende sunt grauide mulieres. Patienter et quiete ne [ni]mia [MS ne mia] gestatione pecus iam perfectum excuciatur [i.e. sent forth, expelled]. Siquidem etiam septimani nasci posset.' (M5)

275–80 *þer-for ... mylk:* 'Ergo neque exerciciis partes illas conuenit fricari, neque pectoralibus fasciis didas constringi; laxamento enim indigent ut et lacte inpleri possint et ne ipsa strictura indignentur.' (M5)

281–85 *But ... mirton:* 'Quomodo viii mense. Cum omni diligentia ac soli[ci]tudine: hoc enim mense plurimum generantur. Quare ab omni nimietate gestationum tranquille sint et cibentur parcius et uentrem fasciis diligenter constrictum suspendant. Etiam et oleo uiridi uel mirtino cutem uentris illiniant.' (M6)

284 *ceprine:* Although both textual families agree here in substance, the manuscript readings *ciroin/ceroin* can only mean a kind of plaster (made from tallow, wax, galbanum, and pitch), not a satisfactory meaning in context. Probably therefore these are errors for some form of 'oyle ciperine' (not cited in MED), deriving either from *ciperus* < Lat. *cyperos,* 'galingale or its root', or from *cipres(se* < Lat. *cypressus*, 'cypress tree', or from *cipre* < Lat. *cypros*, 'henna shrub'. The latter seems the most probable: MED records *ele* (i.e. oil) *of cypro.*

285–93 *And ... brek:* 'Quomodo in nono mense. Fasciande sunt iusum lapsius et subuoluende. Superiores uero partes sub didis amplius stringende ut proximante partu ad inferiora deponatur ut cicius possit exire. Locus etiam ipse laxamentis preparandus encatismatibus [i.e. sitz baths; fomentations] etiam uti et lauacro et pessariis ex adipibus anserinis etiam medulla ceruina [i.e. deer marrow], digito etiam peruncto, os matricis conuenit aperire. Grauide omnes uti non debent uiris si fieri potest .... Nouissimis autem diebus debent se omnino ab hoc usu abstinere. Motus enim importunitate rupto corio [i.e. skin, membrane] humor funditur ....' (M7)

295–301 *And ... secundine:* This section on the secundine or afterbirth is not found in *Non omnes quidem.* It is interesting that the translator thought it necessary to add his own definition here. He may have derived it from an anatomical text although the homely analogy with the egg suggests adaptation to his audience. A somewhat different description is found in *The Nature of Wommen*: 'þe secundine is a skyn þat is of þe veynes and of þe sennes [sinews] of purpyl colour lyk to þe nauel of a schyld whan it is born.' (Green, 'Obstetrical and Gynecological Texts', p. 87)

303–08 *sygnes ... chylde:* Cf. 'Que sunt signa aborsus. Ante le[git]imum tempus parturitionis ratione mamille macriores, frigidior et grauitudo in renibus, humor uarius effunditur et in fine trombus [i.e. clot] uidebitur. Multe etiam aborsorio utuntur ut adultere.' (M8) The ME deviates quite significantly here from *Non omnes quidem*: it censors the reference to adulteresses in particular making use of abortion.

C308 *mysgydynge of her-self:* The only meanings that MED gives for the vbl. n. *misguiding* are 'misrule; false counsel; false administration of laws'; but the meaning 'misconduct' is clear enough from a comparison with D.

309–11 *And ... vse:* D (presumably representing the original translation here) censors Lat.'s casual reference to the desirability of therapeutic abortion in some circumstances: 'Sed si condilomata uel aliqua inpedimenta in orificio matricis mulier habuerit, melius aborsorio exterminare conceptum quam, cum dies partus uenerit, cum exitio mulier pariat.' (M8) C, in contrast, omits this reference to abortion altogether, though the possibility of miscarriage occuring through 'mysgydynge of her-self' glances at it obliquely.

312–23 *Now ... kynde:* 'Unde inpediatur partus ut difficile sit. Primo aut pariens iracunda est aut multum timida uel uerecunda aut primariola. Corpore etiam gracile multum uel pinguis multum aut musculosa aut inbecillis matrix aut in feruore aut aliquibus condilomatibus inpeditur uel orificium coniunctum est aut contortum aut ex parte clusum uel in uicinitate emorroide uel collectiones [i.e. tumours, abcesses] sunt uel in uesica lapis uel in longaone stercorum retentio. Aut infans grande habet caput uel omne corpus uel plura [MS pulcra] membra aut ydrops est uel gibberosus [i.e. hunchbacked] aut languidus aut inflatus uel mortuus aut positus contra naturam.' (M40) Note the abrupt transition to chapter 40 from chapter 8 of *Non omnes quidem.*

326–34 *Whan ... hit:* This is the first occasion on which the Middle English calls on the *Genicia Cleopatrae ad Theodotam*: 'Ad partum iuuandum. Polipodii radicem ei super pedes pone, incoante dolore, etiam mortuum pecus eiciet. Item. Cucumeris agrestis [i.e. wild cucumber] semen quod adhuc in ipsa herba sit et lanam de medio fronte arietis collige et simul repone et cum opus fuerit circa renes aut lumbos habeat. Sed dum pepererit solue ne uulua sequatur.' (MS Laud. Misc. 567, fol. 60)

339–56 *Fyrst ... matryce:* 'Quot scematibus infantes nascuntur. Generaliter iiii modi: in capite, in pedibus, in deuexo [i.e. sloping] iacens aut duplicatus. Specialia quidem scemata sunt plurima. Illi enim qui in capite feruntur aliquando caput in orificio matricis habent, reliquum uero corpus contortum. In capite quidem non descendens aut in priori et non in orificio aut retrorsum caput infigitur aut in auexum [i.e. sloping backwards] se proicit. ... aliquando unam manum foris proicit. Reliqua uero pars intus remanet. Aliquando unum pedem uel alio scemate. Aliquando rectos pedes in orificio habens descendit, manum uero in latere iunctam. Aliquando in priori parte uel retro in orificio infigit. Aliquando unum pedem uel utrosque in rectum foras emittit aut manus similiter supra capite contorto. Aliquando diuisos pedes partibus matricis infigit. Aliquando genua ostendit. Aliquando duplicatus ut sedens naticas ostendit. Aliquando ita duplicatus ut plantas in orificio matricis iunctas inuenias.' (M41)

359–76 *But ... helpe:* A digression. These further recipes for easy deliverance with their strong overtones of superstition and magic are not found in *Non omnes quidem* or the *Genicia Cleopatrae*.

369–72 *Or ... drynk:* Omitted by SC. The ogor-sugor-nogo formula is possibly a corruption of the magical palindrome SATOR-AREPO-TENET-OPERA-ROTAS: see Ernst Darmstaedter, 'Die Sator-Arepo-Formel und ihre Erklärung', *Isis*, 18 (1932), 322–29.

377–80 *3if ... forth:* 'Si in capite descenderit, reliqua parte in latere herente, quid faciendum sit. Inmissa manu obstetrix eum componat manibus, scilicet lateribus iniunctis, ut in orificium reductus descendit.' (M42) Note that in this section all the instructions that were addressed in the Lat. to the *obstetrix* in the third person are addressed directly to the second person.

380–83 *And ... matryce:* 'Quando iunctis pedibus descenderit. Quamquam eum obstetrix adducat sed eum descendere cepit, inmissa manu eius manum teneat et sic adducat ne manus aperiat et lateribus infigat.' (M43)

385–90 *And ... forth:* 'Si grande caput habuerit ut exire non possit. Intrinsecus repellendus est et un[c]tionibus uncto orificio inmissa manu obstetrix eum adducat tenens caput eius adiuuante, et iam conatu suo pariente.' (M44) 'as ys oyle oleve or oyle de bay' and 'in watyre þat fenygrek & lynnesede haue be sodon in' are the ME redactor's expansions.

391–95 *And ... bedde:* 'Si contra naturam positus fuerit. Pariens in lecto iaceat, caput altius habens, et obstetrix immissa manu secundum naturam eum componat et sic adducat. Lectus autem parientis duris stratus sit.' (M45)

396–403 *And ... handys:* 'Si manum proferat, iubemus ut numquam eum obstetrix adducat. .... Iubemus ergo ut humero eius infixis digitis retrorsum reuocetur et componat manus eius iunctis lateribus et apprehenso capite foras eum adducat. Si ambas manus proferat. Duobus humeris eius manus suas ex utraque parte infigens eum retrorsum reuoluet et ut etiam diximus manus lateribus componat et apprehenso capite paulatim adducat.' (M46–47)

404–07 *And ... forth:* 'Si pedes proferat reliquo corpore in aliqua parte inclinato. Sicut diximus obstetrix immissa manu eum componat et sic adducat.' (M48)

408–15 *And ... forth:* 'Si unum pedem eiecerit. Numquam eum adducat nec conetur sed prius digitis ad inguina infantis infixis sursum eum reuocet et post immissa manu pedem alterum corrigat et si fieri potest, manus eius lateribus iungat et apprehensis pedibus foras adducat.' (M49)

411–15 *And ... forth:* 'Si pedes emiserit manu supra capite contorta. Manibus suis inguinibus infixis insursum repellat et compositum ut diximus adducat. Si diuiuos pedes partibus uulue infigatur, inmissa manu obstetrix eos t[e]ntat ad orificium componat et sic adducat.' (M50–51)

416–19 *And ... matryce:* 'Si caput conuersum uel contortum habuerit. Obstetrix inmissa manu corrigat et humeris comprehensum leuiter adducat, ne matrix ipsa quassetur.' (M52) Note that *leuiter* which is perhaps an error for *leniter* is not translated at all by SC, while B has *softely* (the closest to the Lat.), D *a-vysedly* and A *wysly* (probably an attempt to make sense of a D-type reading).

420–25 *And ...hede:* 'Si genua ostendat. Retrorsum repellatur et correptis pedibus adducatur. Si naticas ostendat. Inmissa manu retrorsum eum obstetrix reuocet et plantis in orificium rectis adducat. Si caput et plantas similiter ostendat. Precipimus ut in uulua dis[ip]etur [MS dispietur] et apprehenso capite adducatur.' (M53–55)

425–28 *There ... syk:* This anecdote is not in *Non omnes quidem*, and was possibly introduced by the ME redactor from his personal experience. It is an indication of the problems faced by medieval *obstetrices* and also of the often gloomy prognosis. Here apparently the outcome was relatively successful, but the writer sounds distinctly surprised.

429–34 *And ... all:* 'Si diuiuus iaceat aut supinus uel indentibus [i.e. crooked]. Leuiter obstetrix ... quascumque partes ad orificium propiores habuerit, ipsas teneat et sic adducat, ita tamen ut maxime caput infantis querat et ipsum teneat et foras adducat.' (M56)

435–37 *And ... oper:* 'Si plures uno fuerint et simul se ad orificium contulerint. Sicut diximus in sinum uulue ab obstetrice repellantur et singulatim adducantur.' (M57)

C437–38 *And ... matrice:* Not in D, but cf. Lat.: 'Hec omnia ab obstetrice leniter sine quassatione fiant.' (M57)

439–52 *Yf ... medycyn:* 'Si secund[in]e remanserint. ... statim obstetrix manum sinistram inmittat et quamcumque partem inuenerit teneat et si iam ad fundum recessit, adducat, illa iuuante conatibus suis. Si uero a matrice teneatur, huc et illuc leniter adducat ne indirectum conetur ne matricem simul adducat. .... Si uero clausa in orificium fuerit ut neque manum inmittere possit, utatur omnibus sucis quibus ad feruorem matricis uti solemus ut, hac diligentia relaxata omni strictura, quicquid remanserit mox cadat.' (M10) Here the ME for once follows the Lat. with its construction, 'let þe mydwyffe help'. Note that after using chapters 40–57 of *Non omnes quidem* the ME now reverts to an earlier part of the treatise. In many ways its order is more logical as it brings together all the obstetrical material into one place. In Muscio's *Gynaecia,* from which *Non omnes quidem* derives, this is split between the two parts of the treatise, one on normal and the other on abnormal gynaecological and obstetrical conditions.

453–63 *Aftere ... wyche-crafte:* 'Quomodo umbilicus incidatur. Cum modice infans in terra requieuerit, a uentre digitis iiii scapello aut cultro incidatur; nec supersticioni antiquorum consentiendum est qui uitro uel canna acuta [i.e. sharp reed] uel talibus secabant. ... lana torta uel licio ligabis ne fluxu sanguinis infans periclitetur.' (M15) Note that the material has been somewhat rearranged and that all the ME versions render the gender-neutral *antiquorum* as 'sume olde women' and have introduced a general condemnation of this practice as 'foly & wyche-crafte'.

456 *navyll:* MED does not record the sense 'umbilical cord' but that appears to be the meaning here.

464–70 *And ... mylk:* 'Quando uel unde cibetur infans. Post omnem commotionem, hoc est post viii uel ix horas, talem cibum primum accipiat qui stomachum et uentrem purgare possit et eum nutrire, hoc est, mel modice coctum. Si enim crudum fuerit, inflat. Si uero amplius coctum, constringit. Sic autem detur digito suo nutrix ex melle os eius illiniat uel mulsam tepidam instillet et sic etiam post lac offerat.' (M16)

470–73 *but ... holsame:* 'Cuius lac accipiat infans. Lac maternum non oportet initio dari ... quia maternum ex labore partus et turbore uel purgatione malum est et pingue et indigestibile.' (M17)

472 *purgacyon:* MED does not give the sense that seems appropriate here, 'post-partum flow'. OED does give it, but its earliest example is dated 1555.

474–76 *hyt ... hym:* 'A matre autem oportet infantem nutriri, tamen si solus sit; duobus enim nec sufficit.' (M17) The bizarre suggestion in all the ME versions (except for Sloane, which made the sensible decision to cut it out) is possibly just a misunderstanding of *Non omnes quidem*, which simply says that twins cannot be fed by the mother alone.

477–85 *Tak ... mylk:* 'Qualis queratur nutrix. Adholescens que iam bis peperit, boni etiam coloris, pectus latum habens, hydas neque satis breues neque multum grandes cauernas habentes, animo prudens, non irascibilis, ut toto affectu puerum amet, ebrietatem uitet. Cibum sufficienter sumat. Corpus aliquantulum exerceat. Indigestionem uitet et, si fieri potest, ad uirum non accedat ne usu uenerio purgatio commota superueniat et lac extinguat.' (M18) Note that the Lat. is slightly less strict than the ME in forbidding the wet-nurse sexual activity.

486–90 *And ... corrupcion:* 'Si uero lac nutricis exterminatur, altera queratur nisi restituatur. Antiquitatis etiam supersticio reprobanda est, que pro lactis copia nutricibus ubera animalium sumere in cibo precipiebat. .... Hac enim inportunitate exterminatus stomachus cibos corrupit.' (M18) Note that once again a specific reference to 'svme old women', not merely to 'a superstition of the ancients', is introduced by the ME redactor. Cf. note to 453–63.

487 D *estrayne*, C *estreen:* not in MED but presumably derived from OFr. *estraingne,* 'innards, entrails', although the corresponding Lat. here (*ubera*) might suggest that it means 'udder' (B reads *vddernesse*).

491–94 *sumdell ... lytyll:* 'Bonum enim lac est mediocriter candidum nec subliuidum ... sed mediocriter coagulatum et stillatum leuiter et dilatetur ne se cito diffundat.' (M17)

496–502 *Yf ... norche:* 'Quomodo probamus infantem aptum ad nutriendum. Sique mulier in utero habuit omnibus mensibus, sana fuit, uitali etiam mense sit natus et sit omnibus partibus integer omnesque pori et exitus pateant, uocem solidam habeat mox ut cadit, maxime cum punctus uel molliter digitis pressus uocem emittat, hec omnia integre sensibilitatis signa sunt et pleno tempore natum ostendunt.' (M13)

C500 *twyk:* From OE *twiccian.* According to OED, 'In ME almost entirely displaced by the related *twicchen* TWITCH *v.*1, but still surviving in south-western dial.'

503–05 *There ... powrys:* Not in Lat. or in CS; presumably a thoughtful gloss provided by one of the ME redactors.

506–08 *Let ... harme:* 'Quotiens in die lauetur. Semel et si necessitas euenerit bis. Frequens enim lauacrum capiti eius nocet.' (M21)

509–16 *let ... sekenes:* 'Quotiens lactetur. Frequentius in die lactandus est, modo ex sinistra, modo ex dextera mamma; quotquot sufficiat, semel accipere non potest. ... cum uisus est uelle accipiat, sed ita uero non ante lauacrum uel in lauacro didas trahat, ne ledatur cor eius. Qui enim ante lauacrum uel in ipso lauacro lactantur, scias eos uariis et multis langoribus detineri.' (M22)

520–24 *How ... lothly:* 'Quandiu lactandus est. Post annum et menses sex aut completo biennio, dentibusque iam firmis ut possit solidum cibum commanducare, a lacte separandus est. Ante paucos uero dies paulatim cibum conuenit offerre et rarius ad ditam applicare et nouissime ex toto lac negare et que amara sunt mammis illinire.' (M24)

525–27 *yf ... a-swagyd:* 'Ad lac stringendum. Fortioribus exerciciis et labore cui lac superhabundat utatur.' (M18)

527–28 *let ... schylde:* 'Vt nutrix salsa non comedat. Salsos cibos omnino fugiat quia et puerum corrumpunt et uiuere eius minuunt.' (M19)

533–36 *The ... hert:* 'Signa prefocationis matricis. Retentio spiritus cum omni silentio, nam matrix ad pectus ascendens prefocat mulierem ut quasi mortua iaceat.' (M28)

536–37 *her ... hert:* 'precordia inflantur et thorax grossior fit.' (M28)

538–40 *þe .... lythyll:* 'Vene frontis tumidiores, sudor frigidus per faciem et ceruicem distillat; pulsus nullus inuenitur aut breuissimus.' (M28)

541–46 *oper-whyll ... oute:* 'Aliquando propter silentium similes sunt caducis et apoplecticis et litargicis et que lumbricos habent. Sed hec separantur, quod in his matricis nulla questio precedit et suo loco inueniatur. In prefocatione uero sursum ascendit et que caduce in fine post spasmum saliuas plurimas emittunt et pulsum maiorem habent.' (M28)

546–47 *makyth ... kneys:* Cf. 'aliquando eis manus uel pedes urgentur' (M28) and 'A la fiee si torne isi ensemble, k'ele torne le chief sor les genolz'. (fol. 249va) Fr. goes on to explain (fol. 249vb) that the condition is often the result of sexual frustration.

548–49 *Whan ... syttynge:* 'Cura. Cum ergo ceciderunt, collocentur in cubiculo calido et claro, ita caput altius teneant quasi sedeant.' (M28)

550–51 *þan ...fete:* 'La premereine chose de mecine di ce mal est ke l'on li frie les mains et les piez mesurablement de oile laurin.' (fol. 250ra)

552–53 *makyth ... chynne:* 'et mentum eius frequentius moueatur et sic excitentur et medianis partibus calefactiones admoueas calidis manibus.' (M28)

553–59 *& put ... dovne:* 'et al nes li mete l'on choses de fort odors et de contrarioses, com est de castoire et gabanum et poiz et leine arse et linge drap ars et fumee de peil ars, et de altres choses de fort odor. Oile et oignement doit l'on metre en la naisance ki seient de bon odor, com est yrileon et muceleon, nardileon, ker cestes choses traient la semence et les flors aual.' (fol. 250ra)

C557 *softe of oliues:* Clearly a corruption of D's '& cost & olyuys' and omitted (rightly) as meaningless by S.

558 *yrelyon:* Although all the manuscripts agree on spellings with initial *v-*, the corresponding Fr. is *yrileon* and the Lat. *yrelion.* DMLBS records *irilion*, 'sort of ointment or salve', from Bartholomaeus Anglicus.

  mustelyon, C *mostelion:* Not in MED but corresponds to Fr. *muceleon*, Lat. *mucelion*, glossed as 'oil of musk' by RMLWL, although all the ME manuscripts agree on medial *-t-* rather than *-c-*.

  camelion, C *camelys:* Neither form is found in MED. Although not in Fr., D's reading corresponds to *LSM* 1's *camelion*, probably a form of *chamaemelon*, *camemelon*, 'camomile' (DMLBS). Less likely are corruptions of ME *camedris*, *camedrios*, a medicinal plant, wall germander or hart clover; or of *cameles chaf*, another medicinal plant, probably camel grass.

  nardilion, C *nardileo:* Not in MED; corresponds to Fr. *nardileon*, Lat. *nardilion*, glossed as 'oil of spikenard' by RMLWL.

558–59 *þe sedys:* Aristotle, who 'reduced the role of woman in procreation to that of "prime matter" awaiting the "forming" or "moving" agency of the man's semen' (*Woman Defamed and Woman Defended: An Anthology of Medieval Texts*, ed. by Alcuin Blamires (Oxford: Clarendon Press, 1992), p. 39), taught that 'the female does not contribute any semen to generation' (*De Generatione Animalium* 727b, quoted by Blamires, pp. 40–41). But this text here follows Galen, who knew about the ovaries and taught that the female as well as the male produced 'seed' that was released in coitus through orgasm and that both were necessary for conception. This seed, however, 'must be scantier, colder, and wetter' than man's (*On the Usefulness of the Parts of the Body* II. 301, quoted by Blamires on p. 42). Its retention was a health problem equal to that caused by failure to menstruate. For a brief summary of the ancient and medieval history of this controversy, see Päivi Pahta, *Medieval Embryology in the Vernacular: The Case of 'De Spermate'*, pp. 34–36.

559–60 *And ... fote: Non omnes quidem* suggests cupping, and anointing the vulva.

561–63 *ȝyff ... yn:* 'Si li doint l'on al seir .... le ius del ache ou od le sirup de calament ou od ierapigre ou od le ius del aluisne. .... L'on doit lauer la naisance ... ou de kalament ou de nepite.' (fol. 250ra)

561 *yerapigra, C gerapigra:* Not in MED; corresponds to Fr. *ierapigre*. Lat. *hiera picra* or *pigra* was the term for a purgative whose basic ingredient was aloes.

563–68 *And ... wyket:* 'Justinus li mires commanda a sechier une cuilleree de comin et tribler et doner a boiure et si comanda a prendre l'oint del gopil ou de cheurol et mesler et faire un emplastre et metre desus ou enz od le pessaire. Oribasius commanda a cuire la racine de germandree et fanoil et li uins et le ius chalt geter en la naisance.' (fol. 250rb)

565 *aspaltum, C aspalte* (from S, C reads *aspale*): Neither word is in MED and it is not clear what is meant here. The possibilities are: *aspalthus*, a genus of shrubs with fragrant wood; *aspalathum*, the herb galingale with a ginger-like root; *aspaltum*, which Tony Hunt (*Plant Names of Medieval Britain,* Cambridge: D. S. Brewer, 1989, p. 38, *s. v.)* tentatively identifies with shepherd's purse (*Capsella bursa-pastoris*); or *aspalt*e or *aspaltoun*, native or naturally-occurring asphalt.

569–72 *And ... wombe:* '[S]e la marriz auale a feme quant a eu enfant, si eschaufe l'on mohie, si li mete l'on al uentre en une taie d'orillier.' (fol. 250rb) In Fr. (following *LSM* 1) this is a cure for precipitation, not suffocation, of the uterus.

580 *stermuntacyon, C stermutacion:* Neither MED nor OED records spellings with *-m-*, nor do they give the sense that seems appropriate here of 'a preparation that causes sneezing', which is assigned to *sternutorie*.

581 *fethyr-wort:* Not in MED or OED. There is some doubt about the identification of this plant, which may be either herb paris (*Quartifolium*) or maidenhair fern (*Asplenium trichomanes*). See Hunt, *Plant Names*, p. 124, *s. v.* Gallitricus, and p. 217, *s. v.* Quartifolium.

C581 *struccion:* Possibly a version of Lat. *strution* (see Hunt, *Plant Names*, p. 247, *s. v.* Strutium), which had a variety of ME equivalents including soapwort.

583–84 *The ... plase:* Cf. 'A la fiee se muet la marriz de son liu .... Issi conoist l'on icest mal.' (fol. 250vb)

586–88 *And ... strangelyde:* Cf. 'la dolor tornant a mont al uentre ou el emfle si k'ele ne puet trangloter'. (fol. 250vb)

588 *vom:* This can mean 'vomit' (as A *womyth* and CS *vomet*) but could also be a spelling of 'foam', as B *foome*. The latter seems slightly more likely from the context.

C592 *aspale (mole):* Rather than any of the meanings listed in the note to 565 this may correspond to *aspalax*, a kind of rodent, of which OED gives only one example, dated 1860. Moles were used as an ingredient in medieval medicine: MED gives quotations calling for powder of burnt mole. But also possibly a herb of some kind: Lewis & Short gloss *aspalax* as 'an herb now unknown'.

602–05 *Yf ... yssev:* Cf. 'Ce ke la feme a trop de ses flors .... Cist mals quant il uient del sanc, si estuet la feme seignier, ou en la main ou el braz / por traire le sanc amont, ker li sanc cort touz tens la ou il a eissu.' (fols 248vb-249ra)

605 *ventosse:* OED's earliest example is dated 1500.

605–11 *Good ... drynk:* 'Moult ualt a cest mal a metre la uentose entre les mameles sanz garse, k'ele traie le sanc amont. Le ius del plantein, od la leine carpie, i ualt molt; si la mete l'on dedenz la naisance alques en parfunt; le ius de la iobarbe od le uiez uin, blanc ou roge, est bon a boire. Contre icest mal bon est a prendre leine carpie et moillier en cel ius et lier sor son uentre, et bon est a cuire la racine de la parele en eue ou en uin et boiure le ius.' (fol. 249rb) ME follows Fr., which diverges from *LSM* 1 here.

607 *woll ... scheppe:* M. L. Ryder comments on the 'widespread medicinal use of wool. Hippocrates advocated the use of greasy wool to dress wounds. Wool may help blood to clot, the grease may control drying, and some of the

complex substances it contains may promote growth of new tissue. Wool is unlikely to contain organisms harmful to man, and indeed some secretions of sheepskin are bactericidal', *Sheep and Man* (London: Duckworth, 1983), p. 737. This text possibly specifies wool from a sheep's forehead because that would be finer in quality: 'Medieval wool was ... still predominantly of primitive hairy medium-generalised medium type' (Ryder, p. 476). It was not until after the Middle Ages that there was a 'trend away from the primitive generalised fleece types ... towards modern hairy, medium, short and fine types' (Ryder, p. 477).

613–24 *And ... hym-selfe:* Cf. Fr. 'Se li mals est de cole ... si estuet la feme tel chose que les coles get de li par sueue mecine, com est trifera sarracene, rosate nouuele od escamonie et serup de uioles. Se li mals est d'abondance de flieme ... getez l'en par soeue mecine, com est geralogodion ou feugerole mise en uin ou en ceruoise. Quant li cors est espurgiez des humors dedenz, si estuet reparier as foreines mecines estreignant. Si face l'on la feme boiure eue tieue ou ait enz cuite ... rose ou foille de chaisne ou d'eglentier, et de ronce et d'egremoine et de plantein. Totes ices choses i ualent, ou sengles ou ensemble. Puis li doinst l'on a boiure choses construistes entre uiandes, com est ... poldre de coral, ou pome grenate ... ou de la pome grenate la flor ... et plantein et centoine et sanc de dragon.' (fol. 249ra) *Boiure*, 'to drink', has been misread or misunderstood as 'bathe' in 619.

622 *folefote:* Various identifications are possible, probably because so many plants vaguely resemble foals' feet. See Hunt, *Plant Names,* p. 24, *s. v.* Andrago, p. 37, *s v.* Arus, p. 205, *s. v.* Pes Pulli, p. 151, *s. v.* Jarus.

623 *hertis horne:* Probably a medicinal substance derived from burnt horn, but the term can also refer to various kinds of antler-shaped plants, such as swine's cress (*Coronopus squamatus*) or buck's-horn plantain (*Plantago coronopus*): see Hunt, *Plant Names,* p. 73, *s. v.* Catarian, and p. 194, *s. v.* Ostriagum.

centynody: see Hunt, *Plant Names,* p. 76, *s. v.* Centinodium, for the variety of vernacular names for *centinodium* or *centinodia*.

625–28 *And ... better:* 'et od icestes choses soit le tipsan de orge sechie et cuit et od eue de mara, puis tant ke il crest, et puis quant il est refroidie, si mete l'on l'aisil ouec, s'il colez par un drap, si li doinst l'on a mangier. .... Se il i a racines de plantein od le tipsan, tant ualt mielz.' (fol. 249rb)

628 *And ... in:* 'bone est a boiure l'eu ou les feues soient cuites.' (fol. 249rb)

629–31 *Or ... plastre:* Not in Fr. but present in *LSM* 1 (further proof perhaps that the redactor did not use MS Sloane 3525 itself).

632–35 *tak ... watere:* 'et face l'on poldre des eschales des oes dont li poucin sunt eissu, si doint l'on a boiure a la feme par quatre iourz, chascun iour tant com l'on prendra sus od trois deiz, od eue de mare froide.' (fol. 249va)

C654 *camfory:* D reads *comfyry* so this may be an error, rather than a form of ME *camphre*, camphor (*Camphora laurus*). See Hunt, *Plant Names,* pp. 64–65, *s. v.* Camphora, which also shows *camphre/comfire* confusion.

690 *purge:* The appropriate sense here, 'to begin to menstruate', is not given by MED or OED.

694–96 *Galyen ... bere:* Cf. 'face se seignier de la ueine del pie sor la chiuille, un jor del un pie et altre ior del altre, selonc ice ke ele porra souffrir.' (fol. 247va) This is the only reference to Galen in the ME text: Fr. (following *LSM* 1) does not mention Galen by name here though it does so in the next sentence.

699–706 *tak ... vpward:* Cf. 'Galien dit que la mere erbol triblee et beiue o le uin ualt molt et a la fiee reualt se ele est cuite en eve et beiue en baing, et moult i ualt se ele est uert triblee et liee sor le uentre soz l'omblil, ou se la feme la cuit en un pot, si la mete chaude soz soi, si siee sor une chaiere percee, si se coeure bien de dras, ke la chalor enuoist uers la marriz.' (fol. 247vb) Although the recipes are virtually identical in structure, horehound is not the same as Fr. *mere erbol* (Lat. *artemisia*).

713–18 *For-to... potte:* 'Ad curam conceptionis et menstrua et si matrix ex partu concussa fuerit. Butiri oz v, ysopi oz iii, mirre oz ii, medulle ceruine oz ii, adipis galline oz iii, terebentine oz iii ... mellis quod sufficit, coque in uase fictili nouo et utere.' (M58, fol. 66) The omitted ingredients (Punic wax, hepatic aloes, cassia and rose oil) may have been unidentifiable or too expensive in late medieval England.

718–20 *For ... hooll:* 'Hoc [usa] [MS uasa] est Fabiana Priscilla cum omnes archiatri sine ea [MS archiantresinea] defecissent.' (M58, fol. 66) The ME has misunderstood *Non omnes quidem* here, understandably, as it is corrupt: 'Fabiana Priscilla' is clearly a *medica* or *obstetrix*, not a patient, who succeeds when leading consultants ('court physicians') had failed.

726–31 *Dame ... so:* None of the many recipes in the *Genicia Cleopatrae* for pessaries exactly corresponds to this. Fr. however provides a parallel although it does not attribute the recipe to Cleopatra: 'Se la marriz est si endurcie ke les flors ne puissent uenir o ices mecines, si prenge fiel de tor ou altre fiel et poudre de nitre o le ius d'isope, si mesle l'on ensemble. Si meslez l[e]ine carpie et puis la trecelon ensemble, que le soit alques longue et roide ke l'on la puisse metre en la naissance, et quant ele iert treciee, si la mete l'on enz. Ice a noun pessaire.' (fol. 248ra) *nitre*, (reflected in *a-nutr*e A and *nutre* C) could be easily misread as *mirr(e* (the reading of S and DB).

729 *methill:* MED gives no examples of forms with medial *-th-* rather than *-d-*.

732–35 *A-noþer ... bathynge:* Cf. 'Altre: prengne l'on la rue, mente, / poliol, de chascun une poignee, de la sauge tres ʒ et un plancon de roge colet et tres chief de porez; si les cuise l'on ensemble en un nuef pot, se li doint l'on a boiure et ce apres le baingn.' (fols 248ra–b)

732–34 *A-noþer ... drynk:* Cf. 'si li doinst l'on a boiure et al suer la coeure l'on bien qu'ele sue. Altre esproue: prengne l'on la racine del glaiol et la racine de la guimauue et de luuesche et la nepite, si les cuise l'on en uin, si doint l'on a boiure a la feme.' (fol. 248rb)

738–39 *Or ... navill:* 'taneisie et cerfuoil et altimesie frite od burre, li mete l'on al umblil.' (fol. 248rb)

740–53 *A-noþer ... wynne:* 'Altre: ke li uns li mires fist a la reine de France: gingiure et fueille de lorier et de sauine tribla un petit, si les mit en un pot sor les charbon uis et ele sist sor une sele perciee, ke li funs uint a la nai/ssance, si en ot asez. Mais l'on se doit bien couurir de dras et les cuisses, que li funs uiengne a la naissance. Et ki souent fait iceles estuues, si li besoigne oindre sa naisance dedenz d'uile rosat, k'ele ne s'eschaude de trop. Icest estuue rest bone a faire ... de nepite et de calament et de mente, ou ensemble ou de quel que soit par soi. .... Oignons et porez et eschaloignes et senue et poiure et comin et alz et cerfoil et poisson de eue corant od escherdes et od blanche char, sunt bon a mangier. Li forz uins blans est bons a boiure, se la feme n'a fieure ne dolor del chief.' (fols 248rb–va) *mires* (physician: Lat. *medicus*) at some stage in transmission has presumably been misread as *iuues*.

748 *eschalones*, C *eschalons:* Clearly adapted or derived from Fr. *eschaloignes*; not in MED, which records *scaloun* derived from Anglo-Norman *scalonia* and Anglo-French *scalun, escalone*.

753–55 *Othyre ... moche:* This remark is completely omitted by SC. It corresponds to 'Garses i ualent moult et a hant d'ome' (fol. 248va) (cf. *LSM* 1 'scarificacio et coitus'): the ME has therefore censored these references to cupping, scarification, and sexual intercourse as other cures for the failure to menstruate.

759 *centory:* See Hunt, *Plant Names,* pp. 75–76, *s. v.* Centaurea, for the extraordinary number of vernacular names other than *centaury.*

769 *fy,* C *ffy:* Not in MED or OED but clearly means 'piles' and must be a form (?erroneous) of ME *figis.*

777 *theodoricon euperiston,* C *teodoricon empiston:* RMWL glosses Lat. *theodoricum* as a purgative. These combinations are not recorded by MED but DMLBS cites *theodoricon euperiston* from John Gaddesden and *theodoriton emperiston* from Gilbertus.

780 *as ... before:* That is, at 694–98.

782 *dauck cretyk,* C781 *dauc [creticus]:* From Lat. *daucus creticus,* 'parsnip or carrot'.

   ameos: This unanglicized Latin word is an element in two Latin names that may represent various umbelliferous plants, such as cow parsley, hemlock, and goutweed: see Hunt, *Plant Names,* pp. 20–21, *s. v.* Ameos agreste, Ameos Maior.

C787 *artemesye:* Hunt, *Plant Names,* pp. 36–37, lists three medieval varieties of artemisia or mugwort, but identifies all of them, and their various verncaular names, with *Artemisia vulgaris.*

790 *camedreos:* Hunt tentatively identifies this unanglicized Latin word (which also appears as *camendreos, camedris,* and *camandreos*) with various plants including wall germander and germander speedwell: see *Plant Names,* p. 62, *s. v.* Camedreos.

811–15 *Medycyn ... claryfyed:* 'Prenge l'on del ache et de fenugrec, si les trible l'on bien et destempre od uin, si li doinst l'on a boiure. Altre: prenge l'on / agaric et espaute et la semence de plantein et de sarree, si en face l'on poldre del tot, si li doinst l'on a boiure et od miel cuit.' (fols 250vb–251ra)

816–24 *Hit ... chyld:* Cf. 'La marriz chiet a la fiee aual et ist de son liu et a la fiee ist fors de sa naisance et auient de ce qu'el est trop amoliee la marriz et ist de son liu et par enforcement d'enfanter' (fol. 250rb) and, more particularly, *LSM* 1, which includes material used by ME but not in MS Sloane 3525, explaining why the condition occurs: 'Et hoc contingit propter remollitionem matricis ex nimia frigiditate interius abundante. Huiusmodi autem remollitio et infrigidatio matricis contingit ex frigido aere subintrante per inferius orificium quando s. diu sedet mulier vel super lapidem frigidum vel super aliquid tale' (Hunt, *Anglo-Norman Medecine*, p. 122; cf. Green, 'Liber de Sinthomatibus Mulierum' [52]).

823 *enforsement*, C822 *enforcement:* Not in MED (though it does have *enforcen v.*) but clearly taken from Fr. (see previous note).

825–27 *Þe ... nosse:* Cf. 'S'ele est cheue aual et ne soit eissue, si li mete l'on al nes especes de bone odor.' (fol. 250rb)

828–34 *tak ... oute:* 'prenge l'on amoniac, s'il destempre l'on od le ius d'une puignee d'aluisne, si en oigne l'on le uentre od une pene. Puis prenge l'on une puignee de cassie et altre de rue et altre d'altimesie, si les cuise l'on en uin, si qu'eles deus parz soient escuites et la tierce remaigne, si li doinst l'on a boiure. Eschaufe l'on bien del forment, s'il mete l'on al umblil et al uentre. Quant la marriz est chaue aual et eissue ....' (fol. 250va) The ME is some-what ambiguous and could have been misunderstood as calling for the insertion of this medicine into the womb rather the anointing of the stomach with a feather.

828 *armoniacum*, C827 *aromatum*: From the context, this should be something foul-smelling so C's reading (meaning presumably an aromatic substance) is probably wrong. Neither word however is found in MED, which has only *armoniak* and *aromat*. DMLBS gives three meanings for *ammoniacus*: (a) sal ammoniac; (b) gum obtained from a desert plant; (c) applied to various herbs—also spelt *armoniacum, armoniaca*.

836–37 *put ... place:* 'si la mete l'on enz.' (fol. 250va)

839–44 *There ... pessary:* 'A la fiee auient a la marriz un mauls et une echaufoison ke l'on apele boillement de marriz, ke si est chaude dedenz com s'il i eust breses. En contre icest mal estuet prendre un ʒ et d'opie et de sain d'oue, deus ʒ de la cire de miel de terre, treis ʒ de oile et les albuns des deus oes, et creie et let de feme, si mete l'on ensemble et puis li mete l'on enz od le pessaire.' (fol. 251ra)

845–50 *For ... matryce:* 'A la feme, ke la marriz remaigne en son liu .... Prenge moole de cerf et oint d'oue, et cire rouente et burre, de chascun deux ʒ. Puis prenge l'on fenugrec et linius ... si cuisiez tot ensemble a petit feu, tant ki soient bien cuit, et puis la mete enz od le pessaire. Ker ce ualt a plusors maus ki auienent a la marriz.' (fol. 251ra) ME misunderstands: this is a recipe to ensure that the uterus should stay in its proper place (and that no hardness should remain, an addition omitted by the ME) rather than a recipe for a woman whose uterus is (already) in place.

852–56 *Thys ... euyll:* 'Signa tensionis matricis. Inflatio sub umbilico aliquantulum dura, dolor uentris et renum cum consensu capitis et stomachi, urina inpeditur, uigilie subsecuntur pro punctione. .... Sicut feruorem matricis curabis.' (M29)

857–66 *Thes ... suell:* 'Signa inflationis matricis .... Venter inflatur et digito pressa inflatio cedit et iterum resurgit et si manu percutiatur, sonat ut timpanum. Aliquando cum punctione et tortione uentus huc atque illuc discurrit. Aliquibus inflatio ipsa perseuerat. Aliquibus interdum se ostendit et iterum tollit se. Contingit autem ex frigore uel aborsu uel si trombus sanguinis in orificio remanserit et inde inflatur matrix.' (M30)

864 *abhors:* Cf. 951 *abors:* the forms given by MED are *abort* and the Latinate *aborsum.* Its unfamiliarity perhaps accounts for the even more garbled forms in CS ('an hors') and in A ('horsnes', 'hors').

866–69 *& ... clene:* Cf. 'Sed obstetrix trombum diligenter querat et sine quassatione adducat.' (M30) Note that while *Non omnes quidem* places the responsibility for ensuring that no clots are left in the womb on the midwife, the ME makes the parturient woman responsible for her own welfare.

869–71 *And ... hit:* 'Si uero cronica officiatur, utimur his que in prefocatione uulue. Post epithima, diaspermaton [i.e. drug made from seeds] uel poliarchion [i.e. compound medicine] imponimus et pessarium ex ruta, nitro, pulegio et felle taurino.' (M30)

870 *dyaspermaton,* C868 *diaspermaton:* MED gives only *diaspermaticon* (*s. v. dia- pref.*) but both textual families agree on essentially the same form, without medial *-ic-.* Lewis & Short cite *diaspermaton* from the Greek, meaning 'a drug made with seeds'.

poliarcon, CS (also B) *poliarton:* not in MED but corresponds to Lat. *poliarchon.* Lewis & Short record *polyarchion* as 'a kind of soothing ointment'.

870–73 *Or ... pessary:* 'Item aliud pessarium. Ficus cum granulis et cimini dr. ii [i.e. 2 drachme], afronitri dr. semis [i.e. half a scruple]' (M30) MSS readings *affrotitri* and *affrotiri* are not in MED; they are presumably corruptions of an Anglicized form of Lat. *aphronitrum,* 'efflorescence of saltpetre, sodium carbonate or washing soda'.

874–85 *Be ... blody:* 'Que sunt signa proximi partus. Septimo uel nono mense, grauitudo uteri et renum cum sensu feruoris. Dolor inguinum et lumborum, ipsius et matricis ad inferiorem partem descendentis, orificii apertio et humectatio. Cum uero iam proximat, superiores partes graciliores fiunt et extenduntur loca super pectinem et inguen et frequentis urine desiderium nascitur; inmissoque digito ad magnitudinem oui in orificio inuenitur humor qui fertur primo lentus, postea plurimus et sanguineus.' (M9) This is an abrupt change of subject and the section seems out of place. The section of *Non omnes quidem* used here occurs much earlier than the two chapters (29–30) used from 852–73: possibly it had become displaced in the version used by the ME redactor.

889–94 *The ... pessary:* From the *Genicia Cleopatrae*: 'Signa humorose matricis. Oculorum dolor, caput subcalidum, uertigino, occulta dolent. Cura. Adipem anserinum et butyrum cum aniso trito et cribellato [i.e. sieved] misce, uel linteo mundo subpone.' (C2, fol. 58v)

894–904 *Yf ... vyces:* 'Si ceperit tumor uel uicium in matrice fieri, hec signa sunt. Mamille tume[n]t et duriores [et] sublucide fiunt. Si non curentur, rumpit pus ipsam matricem et fit decursus foras et sic dolor paulatim sedatur. Inde quedam sine filiis sunt et tactum durissimum circa matricem habent, ructant frequenter; quemadmodum ex illo sit [uirum] [MS uerum] tangere nolunt plenasse esse putant. Cura. Suco edere [i.e. ivy] cum modica recente utere et pessum predictum humorose matrici subice que ad omnia uicia eius facit.' (C7, fol. 58v) *swowne* (in one form or another the reading of all the manuscripts except B *dremyn*) is a mistranslation of *ructant* ('belch').

905–10 *The ... swownynge:* 'Signa doloris matricis post partum. Cum se matrix ad stomacum fecerit uehemens nascitur dolor, corpus affligitur, interdum etiam uero in comitiali morbo [i.e. epilepsy] exanimata uidetur, sed hoc distat, quod nec oculi uertuntur nec spumat hernu cum trahuntur, sopor tantum esse uidetur.' (M33)

910–23 *Medycyne ... a-nonne:* 'Cura. Quibus crebro accidit et dolor supra uires fuerit, sanguis emissus prodest. Si paruus sit dolor, cucurbite effugiende sunt inguinibus. Si uero diu iacere aut tacere consueuit, oportet naribus fetorem apponere, et aqua frigida perfundere, aut ex ruta trita, cum melle uel oleo cataplasma natilibus et pube tenus apponere; inter hec perfricare coxas et corpus. Tercio uel quarto die sinapismum [i.e. poultice] lene super uentrem pone ne corpus rubeat. Si uulua exulcerata fuerit, ex rosa et suilla axungia recenti ct oui albugine pessarium apponatur uel cum roseo et rose puluere aut sulfumentum ex sulfure [MS fulfure] fiat et dolorem tollet.' (M33)

924–31 *The ... hete:* 'Signa mole, id est duricie matricis. Hec ualitudo ex precedenti feruore fit. Venter supertenditur ut quasi pregnans uideatur; aliquando carne excrescente, inmisso digito uelut callum sentitur. Aliquando talem altitudinem matrix patitur ut omnis uentus cum duricia lapidem excrescat et reliquum corpus malo colore fastidio tenetur.' (M34) This is the famous 'uterine mole' or tumour, which Soranus was credited with being the first to describe (see *Soranus' Gynecology,* trans. by Owsei Temkin (Baltimore: Johns Hopkins Press, 1956, repr. 1991), III, ix, 36–39). It is interesting that the ME makes use of an entire run of chapters 31–36 in one way or another in this section, but omits M34, which suggests cures for the uterine mole. *Non omnes quidem* notes, 'Some consider this condition incurable', so possibly the ME redactor held that position.

932–37 *The ... marys:* 'Signa duricie in collo matricis. Patens orificium inuenitur punctionibus et doloribus, usum uiri mulier non sustinet. Nam et callosum uidetur quod callum nichil sentiat. Cvra. Vt strictura matricis curetur.' (M32)

938–45 *The ... cyperyn:* 'Signa tumoris matricis. Duricia sub umbilico cum quadam inflatione que cum digito premitus recedit, post iterum se recolligit .... Aliquando pars foris duritia grandis, qua digitis pressa dolorem mulier sentit et cum creuerit duricia reuertitur dolor ad renes et inguen et grauitudo super pecten sentitur.... Cura. Sicut inflationem matricis curamus. Post coque oleo simplici uel ciprino uel telino encolpizamus.' (M31)

946–52 *The ... here:* 'Signa sanguinationis matricis. Lassitudo corporis et tenuitas, fetus color, fastidium etiam aut periculosa ualitudo. .... Aliquando non de matrice sed de sinu mulieris sanguis accurrit. Contigit autem sanguinatio hec ex difficultate partus uel aborsu uel uulnere in matrice, aliqua uenarum corruptione.' (M35)

952–58 *Medycyn ... wolle:* 'Cura omnium. In cubiculo obscuro, lecto firmo pedibus altioribus iaceant. Spongie aqua frigida uel pusca [i.e. dilute vinegar] intincte partibus ipsis apponantur, id est pectini, renibus et inguinibus, et frequenter mutentur, fasciis omnia restringantur, recente etiam facies fomententur, flabellis uentilentur, et caput oleo frigido perungantur et per interualla etiam acetum sorbeant et sucum plantaginis uel uue lupine aut policaris in pessario ponere oportet.' (M35)

959–62 *The ... humors:* 'Signa fluxus sanguinis mulieris. Color fedus, macies corporis, fastidium. Cum ambulat inflatur et tument pedes, aliquando cum dolore et uulnere, aliquando sine dolore et uulnere solus humor fertur. Hec autem ualitudo ex habundantia humoris occurrit.' (M36)

963–71 *Whan ... marys:* 'Cura. Qui fluxus sine dolore et uulnere est, curatur ut sanguinatio matricis .... Quociens autem cum dolore et uulnere fuerit, encolpizamus ex suco alice [i.e. spelt] uel ptisane, relaxatoriis etiam cataplasmatibus, calidis et bonis cibis. Nam his etiam uulnus in feruore positum curatur. Si autem sordidum uulnus fuerit, quod per humorem qui effluit probatur: si feculentus uel limpidus sit, utamur his que disinterici uuluam limpida et sordida curant.' (M36)

974–80 *The ... lytill:* 'Signa lassitudinis uulue. Habundantia menstruorum ut frequenter in mense eueniant cum fastidio uiri et ita ut semen uiri sepe reiciat nec contineat; aborsus eis occurrit et ante legitimum tempus pecus eiciunt et semen quod retineant primo aut secundo aut tercio die excludunt. Aborsum autem secundo aut tercio mense iam formatum sed sine anima et gracile.' (M38) The ME seems to have misunderstood the last sentence of *Non omnes quidem* here, which is merely a description of any foetus aborted in the first trimester.

980–82 *wyche ... blode:* 'Cura. Sicut in sanguinatione matricis et in fluxu ordinauimus sic agatur. Hec enim passio ex fluxu nascitur.' (M38)

984–90 *The ... forme:* 'Signa paralisis matricis. Cum frigore pannosum [i.e. wrinkled, flabby] et solidum orificium ut nec digitum obstetricis sentiat, usum ueneris odit et fugit et si coacta fuerit, non concipit. Ad ambulandum inpeditur; menstrua aut retinentur aut non ordinabiliter eueniunt.' (M39)

990–91 *That ... wondys:* 'Cura. Sanantur sicut que de strictura laborant aut cum dolore purgantur.' (M39)

992–1000 *The ... vrine:* 'Signa inclinate matricis. Matricis collum et orificium in partes iiii inclinantur uel torquetur ante, retro, susum et iusum. Si ad superiores partes digitos obstetricis et aliis signis [*sic*]. Si enim in priori parte et sursum fuerit inclinata, tensio super pectinem sentitur et urina inpeditur. Si uero iusum et retro, stercora cum uentositate exient et cum ingenti difficultate mulier sedet et maxime si ad anum inclinetur.' (M39)

1004 *Medycyn ... euyll: Non omnes quidem* proceeds to prescribe the same treatment as for the uterine mole, which the Middle English redactor apparently chose to omit (see note to 924–31).

1013–1109 *And ... aftyre-byrth:* This section, mainly on apostemes in both men and women, must come from yet another unidentified source. *Non omnes quidem* continues for another two pages in Oxford MS Laud Misc. 567, but the only material that the ME uses from here on is the anecdote about Fabiana Priscilla (see note to 718–20).

1018–19 *herpes omenus,* C *herpesthi omenus:* Norri glosses the ME forms *estiomenus, herpes estiomenus,* as 'gangrene' (Juhani Norri, *Names of Sicknesses in English, 1400–1550: An Exploration of the Lexical Field.* Annales Academiae Scientiarum Fennicae. Dissertationes Humanarum Litterarum 63. Helsinki: Suomalainen Tiedeakademia, 1992, p. 326). MED records the form *herpes estiomenus* from Lanfanc's surgery while Latin dictionaries record forms as varied as *herpes esthiomenus* from Peter of Blois, *herpet' estiomeni* from Gilbertus, and *herpestiomenus* from the Alphita, a medico-botanical glossary. So it is hardly surprising that the vernacular texts are confused too.

1051 *branck vrsyn* (cf. C *braunchis of vrsyn):* An Anglicization of *branca ursina,* for which there are numerous colourful vernacular terms: see Hunt, *Plant Names,* p. 54, *s. v.*

1069 *fyere:* The text proper ends here, though none of the manuscripts indicates this. From here onwards CS diverge completely from DBA.

1109 *aftyre-byrth:* The only occurrence in the text of this word; elsewhere, D uses *secundine.* MED does not record *afterbirth,* while OED's earliest example is dated 1587.

Glossary

Many of the definitions of ME plant names and all Latin botanical names are based on those suggested by Hunt, *Plant Names of Medieval England.*

References are representative rather than exhaustive; all references for any sense or form appearing in D are given first, then all in C. An asterisk before a form or a line reference indicates an emendation. Entries are arranged alphabetically: *y* when used to represent a vowel is treated as vocalic *i; i* when used to represent a consonant is treated as *j; þ* (thorn) is treated as *th; v* when used to represent a vowel is treated as vocalic *u;* 3 (yogh) when used to represent a consonant is treated as *y;* medially as *-gh-,* and occasionally in final position as *z.*

abhors, abors *n.* miscarriage D864, D951, *C863
a-byde *v.* remain D242, C241. **a-bideth, a-bidith, a-bidyth, abydyth, a-bydyth** *v. pr. 3 sg.* D184, C182, C191, C861. **a-bode** *pa. t.* D438. **abyde, a-byde** *v. subj.* D72, C71, C978
abill, abyll *adj.* able, capable D259, C259
abortif, abortyf(fe *n.* an aborted foetus, stillbirth D302, C302. *makyth* ~ causes an abortion D310

abortiff, abortyffe *adj.* born prematurely or dead D293, C292
a-bouth, a-bowte *prep.* around D537, C537, D584
a-bovthe, a-bowte *adv.* around D590, C590
ache *n.* wild celery, smallage (*Apium graveolens*) D790, C791
***affronitri** *n.* aphronitrum, efflorescence of saltpetre D872, C871
a-fore *conj.* before C35
a-fore *adv.* before D406
after, afture *conj.* after D36, C36

afthyre, aftir, afture *prep.* according to D16, D197, C17

aftyre-byrth *n.* afterbirth, placenta D1109

a-gayn(e, a-gaynne, a-yen(s *prep.* against, contrary to D323, D391, D976, C391; opposite, in relation to D262, C262

a-gaynne, a-yen *adv.* again C70, back D409, C409

agaricum *n.* larch agaric (*Polyporus officinalis*) D813, *C812

agrimony, egrimony *n.* agrimony (*Agrimonia eupatoria*) D620, C621

agu *n.* ague, fever D752, C752

aiere, eyere, eyre *n.* atmosphere, climate D516, C514; air D1083

aysell, eysel(l *n.* vinegar D588, D957, C588, C957

ake, hak *v.* ache D97, D170, C97. **a-kith** *pr. 3 sg.* C890. **akyn** *pr. pl.* D854, C854. **ake** *subj.* D803, C802. **akyng(e** *vbl. n.* D808, D890, C584

all *conj.* although D961

a-lich *adv.* alike, similarly C708

all-thow(he *conj.* although D329, D336

ameos *n.* wood-thistle D782, C781

a-myddis *adv.* in the middle C330

a-mys(se *adv.* wrongly, awry D289, C405

an(d, & *conj.* if D94, D253, D492, C492

anacardinum *n.* cashew nut, marking nut (*Semecarpus anacardium, Anacardium orientale*) D776, C775

anckle, ancle, ankyll *n.* ankle D560, D695, C560

aneys, anneys *n.* anise, aniseed D891, C891

angvych, angysch, anguysch, angwish *n.* anguish, pain D85, D91, D584, C584. **anguysch** *pl.* D86

anguisly *adv.* painfully D105

angry, angury *adj.* angry D313, C313

anodir, a-noþer, a-nothyre *adj.* another D182, D685, C685

anoynt, a-noynt(e *v. imp.* anoint, oil D386, D524, C386, C523

a-non(ne, a-noon *adv.* at once, immediately D336, D337, C335

another, a-nother, a-noþer *pron.* another D732, D1015, C732

a-now *adv.* sufficiently D501

antrax *n.* malignant boil or growth D1044, C1043

apetite, appetyt *n.* appetite, desire D809, C809

apium *n.* wild celery, smallage (*Apium graveolens*) C834

apostem(e, a-postem *n.* morbid swelling, inflammation, sore D1027, C1010, C1023. **apostemys** *pl.* D1011, C1011

are, er *conj.* before D721, C640

a-ryse *v.* rise up D543. **a-rysyth** *v. pr. 3 sg.* arises, occurs D102

aristologe *n.* aristolochia, birthwort D788, C788; ~ *longe* D1105

armoniacum *n.* gum ammoniac D828

aromatum *n.* fragrant drug or spice C827

artemesye *n.* artemisia, mugwort (*Artemisia vulgaris*) C787

asafetida *n.* asafoetida (*Ferula foetida*) D1073

aschys, ashes *n. pl.* ashes D795, C794

aspale *n.* kind of rodent, mole C592

aspalte, aspaltum *n.* native asphalt?
D578, C578, C813

assent(yth *v. imp. pl.* concur D460,
C460

a-sonder *adv.* apart C425

a-swage *v.* diminish, reduce (milk
supply) C526. **a-swagyd** *pp.* D527

a-swone *adv.* in a swoon C152

a-svovnynge *ppl. adj.* swooning,
fainting D153

at *prep.* of D883, C882

a-vay *adv.* away D179

a-vyse *v. refl. imp. pl.* take care
D512. **avised, a-vysyd** *ppl. adj.*
wel ~ sensible, sober D480, C481

a-vysydly *adv.* carefully D382

a-wayle *v.* benefit D1073

a-yen(e *see* **a-gayn(e, a-gaynne**

back, bak *n.* back D877, C877.
backys *pl.* backs D96, C96

bad, badde *pa. t.* bade, commanded
D2, D728, C2

bayes *n. pl.* ~ *of lorell, lorere* fruit of
the laurel tree D706, C706

ballyd *adj* bald D42, C42

bareyn, baren *adj.* barren, sterile
D255, C256

barly *n.* barley D625, C625

bathis, bathys *n. pl.* (medicinal)
baths D289, C288

bavme, bawme *n. oyle de, of* ~
balm, balsam, gum of the balsam
tree (*Commiphora opobalsamum*)
D591, C591

be *prep.* by D37, C36

bed(de, bede *n.* bed D392, D395,
C392

beere *n.* bear D1031

beere, bere *v.* bear, produce D33,
C33

befallyth *v. pr. sg.* happens D213.
be-fall *v. impers. subj.* D75

belys *n. pl.* abcesses, boils C1017

be-nethe *adv.* below D276, C275

benys *n. pl.* beans D628, C628

berd(e *n.* beard D43, C43

berthen, bordyn *n.* burden D876,
C876

besy *adj.* busy, occupied D188, C187

besyly *adv.* carefully, diligently
D410, C409

besynesse, bysynes *n.* diligence D14,
C14

best(e *n.* beast, animal D728, C728.
bestis, bestys *pl.* D488, C488

betayne, beteyn *n.* betony D671,
C669

be-twex *prep.* by way of, in the
course of D934

bidith *v. pr. 3 sg.* stays, remains
C542

bynde *v.* constipate, occlude, stop
D468, C467. **bynde** *refl. subj.*
bind, strap D286, C285. **bynde**
imp pl. D328, C327. **bonden,
bounde, bowndyn, bovnde** *pp.*
hampered D948, C948; bound,
strapped D956, C955. **byndynge**
pr. p. clogging D126. **byndyng**
vbl. n. D281

byndynge *n.* binding, bandage D458,
C457. **byndynges, byndyngys** *pl.*
D460, C460

black, blak(e *adj.* black D652, C652,
C1027

bladder(e, bladdyr(e, bladyr(e *n.*
bladder D160, D164, D600, D808,
C159, C166

bladis, bladys *n. pl. leek, lek* ~ leek
shoots? D334, C333

blavnchide *ppl. adj.* blanched D1087

blede, bleede *v. intrans.* bleed D695,
C695; *trans.* (cause to) bleed
D912, C911. **bledyng(e,
bleedynge** *vbl. n.* bleeding,

haemorrhaging D217, D946, C215, C946, C950

bleynes *n. pl.* sores, swellings D1017

blode, blood, bloude *n.* blood D103, C102; sanguine humour D234, C233

boblynge *vbl. n.* rumbling D938

bocchis, boches *n. pl.* boils, abcesses D1016, C1017

body *n.* person D90, C90

boyle *v.* boil D232, C231. **boyle** *imp. pl.* D783, C782

bole, boll(e, boole *n.* bull D728, D871, C728, C870

bollyn *ppl. adj.* swollen, distended C960

*****bollynge** *ppl. adj.* swelling D961

bolnyng(e *vbl. n.* swelling, distention C938, C963

boord, borde *n.* board D457, C457

bor *n.* boar C1031

bordyn *see* **berthen**

born(e, borvne, borvnne *v. pp.* born D274, D329, D464, C274

bothyre, botyr, botthyre, bottyre, butter, buttir, buttyre *n.* butter D715, D739, D846, D892, D1053, C715, C736, C892

botom, bottvm *n.* bottom, base D59, C55

bottok, buttok *n.* buttock D422, C352. **buttokkys** *pl.* D354

bouell, bovell, bowel(l *n.* bowel D156, *D179, D319, C156. **bouellys, bovellys** *pl.* bowels, internal organs D167, D337

bray *v. subj.* cry out, shriek, wail D501

brayn(ne *n.* brain D169, C168

brak(e *v.* expel, eliminate D797, C796

branck vrsyn *n.* bear's breech, hollyhock, sea dock (*Acanthus mollis*) D1051

braunchis, brawnchys *n. pl.* branches, twigs D1051, C1051

breest, brest(e, bryste *n.* breast D509, D511, C509, C536. **brestes, brestis, brestys, brystys** *n. pl.* D45, D278, C44, C278, C303

brek(e *v.* rupture D293, C291. **brekith, brekyth** *v. 3 pr. sg.* D897, C897

bren *n.* bran D832, C831

brenne, bryn(ne *v. imp. pl.* burn D636, D643, C636. **brennynge, brynnynge** *ppl. adj.* burning D841, C840

brent, bront *ppl. adj.* burnt D554, C554

brere, bryere *n.* briar D620, C621

bresyde, brosid *ppl. adj.* bruised, rubbed D1031, C1031

breth(e *n.* breath, breathing D93, D255, C94

brysse *v. subj.* bruise D419. **brosynge** *vbl. n.* bruising C438

brystys *see* **breest**

brode, brood *adj.* broad, wide D287, C286

brosid *see* **bresyde**

brosynge *see* **brysse**

brovessc *n.* broth, soup, stew D1101

burion, bvrione *v.* burgeon, blossom D32, C32

bursa pastoris shepherd's purse, sanguinary D1086

but *conj.* unless D896, C896

cache *v.* catch, grab C440

calament, calamynt(e *n.* calamint, catnip (*Calamintha, Nepeta cataria*) D686, C686, *sirip,* *siruppe of* ~ decoction of calamint D561, C561

calet *n.* foolish woman, harlot D311

camamyll *n.* camomile (*Chamaemelum nobile*) C1072

camedreos, camedrios *n.* wall germander (*Teucrium chamaedrys*) D790, C790

camelys, camelion *n.* wild teasel (*Dipsacus sylvestris*) D558, C558

camfory *n.* camphor (*Camphora laurus*) C654

cancer, cankere, cankyr, kankyr(e *n.* cancer, abcess D1019, D1066, C1019, C1065. **cancvrs** *pl.* D1060

carbuncle, carbunkyll *n.* carbuncle, boil, inflammation D1036, C1036

cas(e *n.* case, situation D94, C94. **casys, *cases** *pl.* D343, C343

cassie, cassye *n.* cassia, cinnamon D830, C829

cast, *caste *v.* vomit up D518, C516. ***casteth, castith** *pr. 3 sg.* expells, throws, sends D168, C167. **cast(e** *subj.* D768, C768. **castyng(e** *pr. p.* D810, C810

castori, castory, castorium, castoryum *n.* castor, dried perineal glands of the beaver D554, D579, D722, C554, C579

cause, cavse, cawse *n.* D152, C151, C155, C174 cause. **causes, causis, causys, cavsys** *pl.* D15, D109, D223, C15, C160

*cawsethe *v. pr. 3 sg.* causes C92

celidony, celydon(y, selidonye *n.* ~ *whyld, weld, whylde, wylde* ~ greater celandine (*Chelidonium majus*) D1038, D1057, C1037–8, C1057

centinodye, centynody *n.* knotgrass, vetch (*Polygonum aviculare*) D623, C623

centory *n.* centaury D759, C759. *lasse, lesse* ~ common or lesser centaury (*Centaurium erythraea*) D781, C780

certayne *adj.* informed D669

certeyn(e *n. in* ~ for certain D29, C29

certified *v. pp.* informed C667

cesith, cesyth, cessith *see* **sece**

chafyng, schavynge *n.* shaving, sliver D360, C360

chaufe *v. pr. pl.* warm by rubbing D231. **chafyd, chavfyde** *pp.* D229, C228. **chafynge, chavfynge** *vbl. n.* D276, D747, C275, C743. **chafe** *v. subj.* C230. **chaf(e, chaffe** *imp pl.* warm by rubbing D552, D567, C553

chambris, chambyrs *n. pl.* compartment (of an organ) D67, C67

change, chaunge *v.* change, alter D659, C659

charge, scharge *v. 1 pres. sg.* charge, enjoin D24, C24

cheken, chekyn, chykyn *n.* chick D296, D654, C296. **checons, chekens** *pl.* C632, C653

chekkys *n. pl.* chicks D632

chepe, schepe, scheppe, sheep, shep *n.* sheep D331, D487, D607, C330, C607. **schepis, schepys, shepis** *poss.* D630, D1070, C630

cheritre, cherytre, chery tre *n.* cherry-tree D670, D766, C669

chese *n.* cheese D642, C642

chyde, child(e, chyld(e, schyld(e *n.* child D7, D70, D115, D360, C6, C426. *with* ~ pregnant D115, C114. **chyldervn** *pl.* D340

childe, chylde *v.* give birth D361, C361. **chyldydde** *pp.* D569.

childynge, chyldynge *vbl. n.* D11, C9, C90

chynnes, chynnys *n. pl.* lacerations, cracks D585, C585

citryn(e *adj.* reddish or brownish yellow D1026, C1026

clappe *v.* pulsate, expand and contract D151. **clappynge** *vbl. n.* D149

clarifyed, claryfyed *ppl. adj.* clarified, freed from impurities D815, C815

clary, *sclarye *n.* the herb. clary (*Salvia pratensis*) D670, C668

cleer, clere *adj.* pure D184; bright D226, C226

clene, clenly *adv.* cleanly D869, C482, C867, completely D190

clensid, clensyd(e, clensydde *v. pp.* cleansed, purified D182, D617, C180, C618

clepid, clepit, clepyd *v. pp.* called D157, D179, D808

clerkis *n. pl.* learned men, scholars C250

cleue *v. pr. pl.* adhere D147, C146. **cleue** *subj.* cling D378, C378

clos(e *adj.* tight D318, C317, C448

coldyrre *adj. comp.* colder D1095

coldith, coldyth *v. pr. 3 sg.* grows cold D241, C241

cole *n.* ~ *lef(e* cabbage leaf D778, C778 *red(e* ~ red cabbage D733, C733. **colys** *pl.* D1057, C1057

colere, colore, colour *n.* choler D229, D613, C613

coleryk *n.* choler C232

coleryk *adj.* choleric C229

colis, colys *n. pl.* coals D578, C578, C739

collys *n. pl.* strained clear broth D1102

*color, colour, colovre, colowre *n.* colour D263, D478, D947, C263

colrage *n.* water-pepper, arse-smart (*Polygonum hydropiper*) D763, C764

comburth *v. pr. 3 sg.* encumbers D150

comenabill, commenabill, commenabyll *adj.* suitable, appropriate D305, D375, D502, C305

comenable, comenabely *adv.* suitably D418, C418

compleccyon, complexion *n.* physical constitution D202, D206, C206

conabill, conuenabyll *adj.* suitable, appropriate D65, C62

conceyle, counseyle *v.* counsel, advise D20, C21

conceyve, conceyue *v.* conceive D37, D266, C78. **conceyuyth** *pr. 3 sg.* D134. **conceyuyd(e, conseyued, conceyvyde, conceyvydde** *pp.* D36, D69, D75, C35, C61. **conceyue, conceyve** *subj.* be conceived D978, C978

congeylynge, congelynge *vbl. n.* congealing, clotting D212, C211

connynge *ppl. adj.* skilfull D357

contrarij, contrary *adj.* contrary, opposite D82, D825, C825

conuenabyll *see* **conabill**

conuenyant, conuenyant *adj.* suitable, likely D266; due, appropriate D497

corall *n.* coral D622, C622

cornis, cornys *n. pl.* cereals D8, C7; seeds, corns D757, C757

corrupcion, corrupcyon *n.* corruption D72, D517, C71. **corrupcions** *pl.* D73, C73

corrupte *adj.* corrupted, rotten D103, C102

cost *n.* costmary (*Chrysanthemum balsamita*) D557

costyf(f *adj.* constipated D483, C483

costifnesse, costyfnes *n.* constipation D807, C807

covrbe *v.* fold, bend D547

cource, cours(e, covrs, cowrs *n.* flow D638, C638, C659; *out of ~* irregularly D224, C223

couer(e, couyre, kyuere *v.* cover D737, D744, D838, C741. **couer(e** *imp. pl.* D893, C893. **coueryd, couyrde** *pp.* covered D704, C704

cowche *v. refl.* lie down D548

cowre *v.* bend C545

creature *n.* created being D2. **creatures, creaturis** *n. pl.* D1, C1

crespes, crispys *n. pl.* kind of pastry D689, C688

creticus, cretyk *see* **dauc(e**

croppis, croppys *n. pl.* any part of a herb except the root D620, D733, C621

cuere *n.* cure D825. **cures, curys** *pl.* D16, C16

cunne, cvnne *v. pl.* know how to D18, C19. **cunnynge** *vbl. n.* C357

cunte *n.* female genitals C48

cuntres, cuntreys *n. pl.* countries D77, C76

curabill *adj.* curable C856

curatyff *adj.* curative, healing D856

curys *see* **cuere**

custom(e *n. of ~* frequently D913, C913

cut(t *see* **kot**

dayesje, daysey, daysy *n.* daisy D686, D1041, C1040. **dayes-jees** *pl.* C686

darnell *n.* tares, cockle (*Lolium temulentum*) D641, C641

dauc(e, dauck, dauk *n.* parsnip, carrot D790, C791; *~ creticus, cretyk* Cretan carrot (*Athamanta cretensis*) D782, C781

ded *see* **do**

ded(e *adj.* dead D152, C151, C307

dedeuyt, dedyut, deduit *n.* (sexual) pleasure D79, D484, D901

deede *n. ~ of hire naturall lykynge* her act of sexual intercourse C79–80; *the naturall ~* C934

deer(e, der(e *n.* deer D290, D593, C288, C593

defaut(e, defautt, defavte, defawte *n.* D89, D97, D122, D214, C89, C172; failure, lack D771, C771

defey, defie, defy(e *v.* digest D123, D188, C120, C489. **defieth, defyet(h** *pr. 3 sg.* D121, D125, C119, C122. **defey, defye** *pr. pl.* D118, C116. **defyed(e** *pp.* D182, C180

dey, dye *v.* die D112, C109

dele *v. ~ naturally* have intercourse C986. **dele** *v. subj.* act C438

deliuer, delyuere *v.* deliver, cause to give birth D336, C334. **deliuered, deliuerid, delyuerd(e, delyuyrd** *pp.* delivered D333, D443, D906, C332, C442

deliueraunce, delyuerance, diliueraunce *n.* release, delivery (in childbirth) D98, D134, C97, C325

descendit *v. pr. 3 sg.* descends, passes down D183

despite, dyspyte *n.* spitefulness D25, C25

devly *adv.* duly D164

dew, due *adv.* proper D394, C394

dewery, drewery, drewry, drwere
n. love-making, sex D250, D901,
D976, D987

diamargariton, dyamergariton *n.*
drug made from pearls D364,
C364

diaspermaton, dyaspermaton *n.*
drug made from seeds D870, C868

dyetynge *vbl. n.* eating D1097

discreet *adj.* wise, sensible C90

**dysese, disesse, dishese, dysesse,
dissese** *n.* disease D21, D214,
D942, C22. discomfort D304,
C165. **desesys, dysessys, dishesis**
pl. D167, D280, C279

dysesyth *v. pr. sg.* diseases D85.
deshese, dysesyn, dishese *pl.*
D87, C85, C86

disioyne, dysyonne *v. subj.* separate
D412, C412

disioynt, dysioynte *v.* spread out
D397, C397.*dysioynted,
dysiontyde** *pp.* D382, C383

display, dysplay *v. imp. pl.* separate
D424, C424

disport *n.* play D291

dispose *v. refl. subj.* conduct oneself
C483. ~ ... *here body naturally*
have sexual intercourse C290

distroyde *v. pp.* destroyed D128

dystrovbelyd *v. pp.* troubled D313

disturbelyde *v. pp.* disturbed D997

disturbyd, dysturbyde *v. pp.*
disturbed, troubled D317, C316,
C998

dytayn(e *n.* dittany D363, C363

diuers(e, dyuers(e *adj.* diverse,
varied D15, C10, C160, C312

diuersite, dyuersyte *n.* difference
D41, D44, C41; distinction D541.
diuersites, dyuersyteys *n. pl.*
D40, C40

do *v.* ~ *myn ententyffe bysynes,
ententif besynesse,* do my utmost
D14, C14. *haw* ~ have (sexual)
dealings D901. **ded(e** *pa. t.* did
D740, D903. **do(nne** *pp.* D191,
put, applied C896

docke, dok *n.* dock D610, C610

dong(e, dunge *n.* dung D630, D1041,
C630, C648

dovys, dowes *n. poss.* dove's
D1041, C1040

douter, dowhter *n.* daughter D726,
C726

drame *n.* dram, drachm (1/8 oz.)
D581. **drammys** *pl.* D363

drav, drawe *v.* translate D14, C14;
pull D411, C441; ~ *breth* breathe
C150. **drawith, dravth** *pr. 3 sg.*
moves D288, C286. **draw, drawe,
dravn** *pr. pl.* D148, gather C192,
move, sink D193. **drav, draw(e,
drawhith** *imp. pl.* D402, D437,
D640, C640, strain C847. **drawe**
subj. C438. **drawen, drawyn** *pp.*
D22, C22. **dravynge** *vbl. n.* D93

drede *v.* dread, fear D137. **dredynge**
pres. p. D27, C27

dresse *v.* arrange D79, C79. **dressid**
pp. arranged, composed C432.
dresse *imp. pl.* D379, C379

drewery, drewry, drwere *see*
dewery

dryed *ppl. adj.* dried up, desiccated
D128

drynck, drynk *n.* drink, drinking
D228, D482, C227. **drynkes,
drynkys, drynkis** *n. pl.* drinks
D621, D722, C622, C722

drynck, drynk(e *v.* drink D707,
D753, C752, C1004

dronklew *adj.* given to drunkenness
D481

dropsy *n.* dropsy D112, C109

duellyth, dwellith *v. pr. 3 sg.* abides,
exists D845, C845

ease, ese, esse *n.* comfort, relief
D648, D919, C648
ebrose *n.* a laxative C614
ech(e *pron.* each D624, C624
eche *adj.* each C633
eg(ge *n.* egg D296, C295, C632.
eggis, eggys *pl.* D653, C1005
egyre, egre *adj.* sharp, stinging,
strong D838, C837
egrimony *see* **agrimony**
eyen, jen, yes *n. pl.* eyes D890,
C890, C908
eyere, eyre *see* aiere
eysel(l *n. see* **aysell**
elys *n. pl.* eels D1104
elys, ell(is, ellys, els *adv.* else D48,
D308, D317, C272, C336
emerawdys, emeroydys *n. pl.*
haemorrhoids D217, C216
emplaustre, enplastire *n.* plaster,
salve-like preparation D1030,
C1030. **emplastris, emplaustrys**
n. pl. D966, C965
empostem *n.* aposteme, abcess
D1039. **empostemys** *pl.* C1051
encens(e *n.* incense D804, C802
encombrith, encomburth *v. pr. 3 sg.*
burdens D489, C488
endewere *v.* endure D911
endured, induerde *ppl. adj.*
toughened, hardened D727, C727
enforce *v. refl.* exert, force C442.
enforsith, enforsyth *pr. 3 sg.*
causes D198, C198
enforcement, enforsement *n.* force,
violence D823, C822
engendyrde, engendrid,
engendryde *v. pp.* engendered,
conceived D7, D35, C6
engendrure *n.* C11 reproduction

Englysch, Inglish, Inglysh *n.*
English (language) D15, C15, C23
eny, ony *adj.* any D19, C67
enterlacyde, enterlasyd *ppl. adj.*
crisscrossed D56, C53
entermet *v. refl. subj.* involve oneself
D291, ~ ... *of* take part in D483
ententif, ententyffe *adj.* attentive,
careful D14, C14
entyre, entre *v.* enter D518, C515
entre *n.* entrance, opening D58
epithym(e *n.* epithymum, thyme
dodder (*Cuscuta epithymum*)
D870, C868
er *see* **are**
erbe, herb(e *n.* pasture D330, C329;
herb, plant D700, D1092. **erbis,**
erbys, herbys *n. pl.* D8, D783, C7
eschalons, eschalones *n. pl.*
scallions, onions D748, C748
ese, esse *n. see* **ease**
ese *v. imp. pl.* relieve C394
esy *adj.* moderate, gentle D848,
C849; easy D502, C502;
convenient C434. *esyest* *superl.*
D434
esily, esyli, esyly, esly *adv.*
comfortably D106, D271, C104,
C392, C432
esporgymente, espurgement *n.*
purgation, purification D34, C34
estorax *n.* styrax, the gum resin
C708. *see also* **storak**
estrayne, estreen *n.* innards, udder
D487, C487
euen, euyn, even, evyn *adv.* exactly
D62, D262, C59; equally D1007,
C1007, ~ *foorth, forth* straight out
D446, C446
euil(l, euyll *n.* ill, ailment D598,
C321, C597, C863. **euelys, evillys,**
euylys, euyls *n. pl.* D29, D323,
C30, C850

euyll, evyll *adj.* evil, ill D199, D255

fayle *v. trans. pr. pl.* cease to have D247. **faylyth, failith** *intr. 3 sg.* fails, ceases D487, C487. *****fayllyd, faylid** *pp.* proved unproductive D654, C653. **failyng, faylynge, fayllynge** *vbl. n.* failing, ceasing D204, D664, C204, C663

fair(e, fayere, fayre, feyre *adj.* fair D687, C687, good-quality D1035, C1035; pleasant D548

fayre, faire *adv.* carefully, thoroughly D795, C549, C794

fall(e *v.* happen, befall D27, C27. **fallyth, fallyth, fallit(h** *3 sg.* falls D38, D72, C37, C71, *impers.* befalls, occurs D205, C9; **fall(e, fallyn, fallvn** *pl.* D11, D131, D167, C130. **fall(e** *subj.* D24, C24. **falle** *pp.* D251, C252

fastenyth *v. pr. 3 sg.* attaches D349. **fastenyde, fastnyd** *pp.* stuck D162, attached C444

fastid *pp.* attached C161

fawte *n.* lack C356

febill, febyll, febull *adj.* feeble, weak D9, D559, C8

febillith *v. pr. 3 sg.* enfeebles, weakens C240

fedir, fethyre *n.* feather D551, C551. **(f)federis, fetherys, fethyrs** *pl.* feathers D555, D594, C555, C593

feeld, felde *n.* field D750, C750. **feldys** *pl.* D1098

feer, fier, fire, fyere *n.* fire D848, C849, C1067; ~ *of helle* kind of skin complaint D1010, C1010

fel(e *v.* feel, sense D986, C986. **felyth(e, felith** *pr. 3 sg.* experiences D304, D306, C305

felle, fill *v. refl.* fill D279, C278

female, femall, femell *adj.* female D83, C83, C488. **femalys** *pl.* D488

fenell, ffenell *n.* fennel (*Foeniculum vulgare*) D790, C791

fenigrek, fenygrek, ffenygrek *n.* fenugreek (*Trigonella foenum-graecum*) D364, D712, C363, C847

feruent, fervent, ferwent *adj.* burning D840, D925, C839, C924

fervoor *n.* heat, fever D968

ferste, firste, fyrst(e *adj.* first D41, D87, C41, C257

ferste, firste, fyrst(e, furste *adv.* first D40, D53, D86, D377, C40, C341, C665

fesawnt *n.* pheasant D1097

festre, fystere *n.* festering sore, cancer D1066, C1064

fethyrfoy, ffethirfoye *n.* feverfew (*Chrysanthemum parthenium*) D738, C735

fethirwort, fethyr-wort *n.* featherwort (see note) D581, C580

feuir, feuyre *n.* fever D752, C752. **feavrys** *pl.* D854

feve *pn.* few D248

ffy, fy *n.* piles D769, C769

fyfte *adj.* fifth C48

fygge *n.* fig D660, C660. **fygges, fyggis** *pl.* D872, C871

fynger(e, fyngyre *n.* finger D397, D469, C881. **fyngers, fyngyrs, fyngres, fyngris** *n. pl.* fingers D458, D596, C458, C468

flank(e *n.* thigh D913, C955. **flankis** *n. pl.* C912

flappe *v.* move to and fro C149. **flappynge** *vbl. n.* C148

fleche, flesch(e, flesh *n.* flesh D750, D927, D928, C750

fflegmon, flegmon *n.* inflammation caused by excess of the humour of blood D1017, C1017

flevme, flewm(e *n.* flegm D234, D1020, D1023, C233, C615

flex *n.* flax D566

flouyre, flour, flovyre, flowr(e *n.* menstrual flow D218, D771, D773, D988, C231. **floures, flouris, flourys, flours, flovrys, flowres, flowris. flowrys** *n. pl.* D35, D38, D172, D223, C37, C89, C100, C113, C114, C115, C223 menstruation. *white ~* discharge C1070

flour, flowere *n.* flour D687, C687

floure *v.* flower D33, C32

flowes *n. pl.* flows C854

folefote, fole-fote *n.* coltsfoot (*Tussilago farfara*, see note) D622, C622

foly *n.* foolishness D461, C460

fore-nemydde *ppl. adj.* previously named D1102

forgeth, forkys, fourches, fourgez, fowrgeȝ *n. pl.* crotch, forked party of the body D409, D955, C409, C943, C954

forme *n. in dew, due ~* properly D990, C990

forme *v.* form, shape D64. **formyd(e, fourmed** *pp.* D54, D979, C61, C980

forowed *n.* forehead D943

forsayde, forseyde *ppl. adj.* aforesaid D161, D1103

forsse *v.* make an effort D443

foule, fovlle *n.* fowl, bird D1098, D1102. **foulys, fovlys, ffowlis** *n. pl.* D750, D1099, C750

foule, fowle *adj.* foul, disgusting D969, C967

foule, fouly, fowll *adv.* foully, disgustingly D866, D970, C865, C968

fourte *adj.* fourth C45

franckensensse *n.* frankincense D1070

Frenche, Frensh *n.* French (language) D48, C18

frete *v. imp. pl.* rub C576

fretyde, frettid *ppl. adj.* criss-crossed D56, C53

froyte, frute *n.* fruit D33, C33

front(e, frownt *n.* forehead D42, D331, C41, C330, C538

frot(e *v. imp. pl.* rub D550, D917

fulfyll *v. intrans.* mature, reach fufilment D252

fume, ffume *n.* fume, miasma D169, C167; smoke D704, C784

fumygacyon *n.* subfumigation D556. **fumigacions, fumigacyons** *pl.* D745, C742

gadrith *v. pr. 3 sg.* gathers, accumulates C226. **gadderyde, gaderid, gaderyde** *pp.* collected D160, D227, C160

galbanum *n.* galbanum (gum resin) D554, C554

gall(e *n.* gall-bladder D728, C728

gencian, gencyan *n. longe ~* ?gentian (*Gentiana amarella*) D788, C788–89

gendrynge *vbl. n.* reproducing D12

geralagodion, yeralogodyon *n.* purgative medicine similar to hiera picra D616, C615

gerapigra, yerapigra *n.* hiera picra, purgative of which the basic ingredient was aloes D561, C561

geve, gyfe, ȝeue, *v.* give D509, D613, D681. **gyf** *pr. pl.* D486. **gif, gyf(fe, ȝef(f, ȝif(f, ȝiffe, ȝyf(f** *v. imp. pl.*

D363, D366, D368, D372, D561, D611, D617, D618, C613, C660.

gyve *subj.* D470. *see also* **yeue**

gynger(e *n.* ginger (*Zingiber officinalis*) D740, C737

girdill, gyrdill *n.* girdle, belt D287, C286

girdith *v. pr. 3 sg.* girds, binds C277. **gyrde** *subj.* D278. **gerde, gyrde** *imp. pl.* D373, C370. **gyrdynge** *vbl. n.* C279

gladyn *n.* gladden, yellow flag iris (*Iris pseudacorus*) D1081

gladyoll *n.* yellow flag iris D735

glett *n.* flegm, corruption C810

goldys clot ?common burdock D1091

goos, gosse *n.* goose D630, C630

got *v. pr. sg.* goes, passes D504. **goeng, goyng(e** *vbl. n.* walking D270, D277, C269, C988

gote, got(t, gotte *n.* goat D290, D565, D642, C288, C642. **gotis, gottys** *poss.* D750, C750

govte, gowt(e *n.* gout D541, D542, C541

graynes, greynes *n. pl.* grains, seeds D872, C871

grece, gres(se *n.* grease D564, D630, C564, C630

Greek, Grek *n.* Greek (language) D17, C18

grene *adj.* green D576, C576

grete, grett *adj.* large D282, C281

gretnes(se *n.* size D883, C882

grevans, greuaunce, grevaunce, grewance, grewans *n.* pain, discomfort D935, D942, D963, C934, C941

greve *v.* hurt, harm D518, C515

grevys *n. pl.* sores? D585

grope, groppe *v.* feel, search D899, C898

grosnesse *n.* thickness D212

grovyth, groweth, growith, growth *v. pr. 3 sg.* grows D327, D330, C329, C330

habundaunte, habvndant *adj.* abundant, plentiful D526, C525

***hacched, hacchid** *v. pp.* hatched D632, C632

hak *see* **ake**

half(f *n. to the ~* i.e. to half the quantity D831, C830–31

hange, honge *v. imp. pl.* hang, suspend D637, D639, C639

hangynge, hengyng, hongynge *ppl. adj.* pendulous D46, D1034, C45, C1034

hard(e, herde *adj.* hard, firm D392, C392, difficult C950, hardened D711

hardyd(e *ppl. adj.* hardened D727, C711

hardnes(se *n.* hardening D924, C924

harme *n.* arm D603

hare, harre, here, hir(e *poss. adj.* her D92, D874, D877, C874, C876

hart, hert(e *n.* heart D92, D146, D947, C92

hasty *adj.* rapid, swift C364

hastyly *adv.* rapidly, swiftly D226

hasull *n.* hazel D366

hate *v.* hate D986, C986. **hat, *hateth, hatith, hatyth** *pr. 3 sg.* D197, D975, C196, C975

haw *v.* have D901. **hawe** *pr. pl.* D1094

hed(e *n.* head D169, C167. **hedis, hedys** *pl.* D733, C733

heer-aftir, her-after, hereafture, hire-aftir, here-aftere, here-aftyre *adv.* later D39, D99, D246, C38, C219, C258

heyhofe, heyhow *n.* ground ivy (*Glechoma hederacea*) D675, C673

hele *n.* health, welfare D26, C26

hele, helyn, hell *v.* heal D937, D1037, C936, C980. **helyd** *pp.* D1064, C1063

helpe, helpyn *v.* help D981, C981. **holp, holpe(n, holpyn, holpon, j-holpyn** *pp.* helped, assisted D94, D110, D144, D245, D888, C94, C107, C887. **helpynge** *pres. p.* D16, C16

hengyng *ppl. adj. see* **hangynge**

hen(ne *n.* hen D653, D693, C653. **hennys**. *poss.* D640, C640

her(e *n.* hair D651, C650

herb(e, herbys *see* **erbe**

here *poss. adj.* their D15, C15

herere, hier, hyer(e *adj. comp.* higher D80, D953, C80, C953

herpesethi omenus, herpes omenus kind of abcess (see note) D1018–19, C1018–19

hertis *n. poss. ~ horn(e* hart ' s horn (see note) D623, C623

het(e *v. imp. pl.* heat D650, C650

heuynesse, hevynes *n.* heaviness, weight D876, D943, C876

hye *n. an ~* on high, aloft C393

hie, hy(e *adv.* high, elevated D392, C549, C586

hier, hyer(e *see* **herere**

hindforth *adv.* towards the back C999

hype, hyppe *n.* hip D80, C80. **hipes, hyppys** *pl.* D877, C877

hog(ge *n.* hog, swine D846, C970

hol(e, hool(l *adj.* whole, healed D220, D720, C597, C720. *~ fote* web-footed D1099

hold(e *v.* D64, D66, C60 hold. **hold(e** *subj.* D396, D711, C396, C711.

hold(yth *imp. pl.* D432, D594.

holden, holdyn, holdon *v. pp.* held, retained D444, D705, C444, possessed D931, C930; **holdvnne** withheld D208

holsame, holsome, holsum *adj.* wholesome, healthy D473, D495, C471

hony *n.* honey D466, C466

hore hound, horhond, horhownd(e *n.* horehound D699, D790, C699, C790

horsdonge, hors dunge *n.* horse manure D648, C648

hosbande, hosbonde *n.* husband D81, D257

hote *n.* heat D73

hote *adj.* hot D4, C3

howr, ovyre *n.* hour D464, C464

humore, humour, humvre *n.* (Galenic) humour D129; swelling, (sac of) fluid D883, C882. **humorys, humors, humoures, humours** *n. pl.* D38, D199, C37, C125

jen *see* **eyen**

ille, ylle *adj.* evil, bad C199, C256

incurabyll, in-curabyll(e *adj.* incurable D112, D244, D258, *see also* **oncurabill**

induerde *see* **endured**

j-now, jnowh *adv.* enough D188, C188

inpressith *v. pr. 3 sg.* presses on C587

***yrelion, *yrelyon** *n.* irelion D558, C558

jsop(e, ysop *n.* hyssop D368, D715, C368, C729

issew, jssew, issu, yssev *n.* exit D166, C167, C218, C774

yuery, yvery *n.* ivory D360, C360

yuy, ivy *n.* ivy D902, C900
yeralogodyon *see* **geralagodion**
yerapigra *see* **gerapigra**
iocvnde, jocond *adj.* cheerful D264,
   C264
joyce, joyse, juce, jus(e, jusse *n.*
   juice D562, D608, D687, D966,
   D1037, C562, C608
yoyfull, joyefull *adj.* joyful,
   lighthearted D124, C122
yoyne, joyne *v. imp. pl.* join D414,
   C414. **yoynyde, yonyde, joyned,**
   joynyd(e *pp.* joined D93, D161,
   D195, D355, C193
*iointis, joyntis *n. pl.* joints D536,
   C536
joyntly, yontly *adv.* jointly D342,
   D349, C343
jussell *n.* eggs or fish-roe cooked in
   broth D1101

kankyr *see* **canker**
keende, kende, kynde *n.* nature
   D142, C142, C254. *a-gaynne,*
   a-yens ~ unnaturally D391, C322,
   C391
keendely, kendly, kyndly *adj.*
   natural D242, D243, C242
kepe *v.* care for D267, C267. **kepe**
   subj. D268, C268
kycumbres *n. pl.* cucumbers D913,
   C912
kydde *n.* kid D1099. **kyddis, kyddys**
   poss. D750, C750
kyuere *see* **couer**
knees, kneys *n. pl.* knees D354,
   C352
knov, know(e *v.* know D16, C16,
   C225. **knowith, knowyth, knovth**
   pr. 3 sg. D90, D511, C91. **knov,**
   knowe *pr. pl.* D268, C267. **know**
   pp. D225

kot, cut *v.* cut D461, C461. **cut, kit,**
   kyt *imp. pl.* D372, D460, C459.
   cut(t *pp.* D456, C456
kow *n.* cow D487

labour, labure *n.* labour, toil D118,
   C116
laboureth, labure *v. pr. 3 pl.* labour,
   toil D118, C115
large *at* ~ free D283, C282
lasse, lesse *n.* less D202, C202
laste *v. subj.* last, persist C911
lawnce *v. imp. pl.* lance D1034.
   launcyd *pp.* C1034
lauy, lavy *adj.* unruly D256, C257
laxatiffis, laxatifiis, laxatiuis,
   laxatiuys *n. pl.* laxatives D614,
   D966, C613, C614
laxatiffis, laxatiuis, laxatyuys *adj.*
   pl. laxative D722, D1029, C1029
led(de *n.* lead D947, C947
leddyr *n.* leather, skin D55
leek, lek *n.* leek D334, C333. **lekys** *n.*
   pl. leeks D733, C733
leen, lene *adj.* lean, emaciated D207,
   D960, C207
legges, leggis, leggys *n. pl.* legs. D46,
   D381, C46, C381, C917
ley *v.* lay D702, C702. **lay, ley** *imp.*
   pl. lay D457, D804, C456. **layde**
   pp. D568. **ley** *subj.* D379
lese *v.* lose D113, C168. **lesith,**
   lesyth *pr. 3 sg.* D242, C241. **lese**
   pr. pl. D114, C113
lesse *v.* lessen, reduce D1077. **lesse**
   subj. *D912, C771
let(te *v¹* *imp. pl.* ~ ... *blode* (cause to)
   bleed D779, C779
lette *v²* hinder, prevent D312, C312.
   lettyd *pp.* D108, C106
lettynge *vbl. n.* hindrance D324.
   lettyngis *n. pl.* C324

lettyrde, lettrid *ppl. adj.* learned, literate D20, C20

letuse *n.* lettuce D1086

leue *v¹ subj.* live C95

leue *v²* leave, abandon D754

leuis, leuys, levys *n. pl.* leaves D660, C660, C737

lewke *adj.* lukewarm, tepid C620

licour, lyqure *n.* liquid D1047, C1046

ly(e *n.* lye, detergent D794, D795, C794

lye, ley *v.* lie D391, C80. **lyes, lyeth, lyth** *pr 3 sg,* D84, D161, C84, *C296. **lye, lyyth, lyth** *pr. pl.* D61, D163, C162. **ley, ly** *subj.* D80, D379. **lyinge** *pres. p.* C55

lyf(fe *n.* life D186, C184

lyfly *adj.* full of life D502, C501

lyfte *adj.* left D62, C58

lightly, lyghtly, ly3thly, lytely, lythely *adv.* easily D273, D473, D493, C272, C492; ?carelessly D447, C446

lignum aloe *n.* the drug aloes, aloes wood D557, C557

lykyng *vbl. n.* naturall ~ (sexual) pleasure C976

lyly *n.* lily D1055, C1055

lynen, lynyn *adj.* linen D644, C644

lyne-seed(e, lynnesede, lynsed(e, lynseed *n.* seed of flax, linseed D389, D567, D712, C388, C641, C656

lynett, lynt *n.* lint D1035, C1035

lyst, luste *v. pr. pl.* like D1094, D1096

litarge, lytargion *n.* litharge, lead monoxide D1048, C1047

lythill, litill, lityll, lytyll, *adj.* little D215, D296, D298, C213

lythy(l, litill, lytyll *adv. a ~, but ~* a little way, for a little while D453, D455, C453; scantily D540

liuer, lyver, lyuer(e, lyuyre *n.* liver D122, D146, C120, C146, C187

longaon *n.* rectum D157, C156

longys, lunges, lungys *n. pl.* lungs D147, C146, C148

longe *v. pl.* belong, appertain C11. **longith** *pr. 3 sg.* D253, C253. **longyng** *pres. p.* D12

lorell *n.* laurel, bay C676

lorer(e *n.* laurel, bay D677, D741

loth(e *v.* dislike C524, disgust D525

lothly *adj.* unpleasant D524

louach(e *n.* lovage (*Levisticum officinale*) D736, D1092

low(e *adv.* low down D816, C816

luck-warme *adj.* luke-warm D619

luste *n.* desire D773, C773

mayde *n.* girl, virgin D250, C251

mayden, maydyn *n.* maiden, girl D249, C1070. ~ *schyld* female child D70. **maydenys, maydyns** *pl.* D123, C121

maistris, mastrys *n. pl* masters, experts D17, C17

makere *n.* maker, creator D32

malecoly, malencoly, melancholy *n.* black bile D213, C213, C1026

maledy *n.* malady, disease D773, C773. **maladyes, maledies, maledyes.** *pl.* D15, D21, C15, C21

malov *n.* mallow D566. **malovys, malovs, malows, malues, malwes, malwis** *n. pl.* mallows D686, D796, D966, C686, C795, C965

maris, maryce, marys *n.* womb, uterus D51, D87, D1073

matier, matyre, mature *n.* matter D4, D5, C3

matrice, matryce, matrys(se *n.*
womb, uterus D54, D84, D252,
D586, C50

meche, moche *adv. for as* ~ for as
much D9, C8

mechill, mekill, mochyll *adj.* much
D208, C207, C541

mede *n.* mead D724, C724

**medecyn, medycyn(e, medycynne,
medyson** *n.* medicine D110,
D257, D365, D891, C134, C963.
**medicines, medicynes,
medycines, medycynys,
medycyns** *pl.* D220, D245, C107,
C219, C325

medyll *v. pr. pl.* mix D231. **medill,
medyll, methill** *imp. pl.* D331,
D565, D729, C565, C646. **medyll**
subj. mingle, combine C230.
medelid *pp.* C1040

**medill bark, myddilbark, myddyll
bark** *n.* middle of the bark D766,
C668, C765–6

megyr, megre *adj.* slight, slender
D315, C314

mekyll, mochyll, mokyll *adv.* much
D120, D207, D261, C118

membir *n.* part of the body C46.
**membyrs, membres, membris,
membrys** *pl.* D12, D186, D322,
C11

men *adj.* ~ *tyme* (in the) meantime
D683

menewhile, mene whyle *adv.*
meanwhile D395, C681

menstrual, menstrualis *adj.*
menstrual, monthly D201, C200

menge *v.* mix, mingle D843. **menge**
v. imp. pl. C842

mengyll *v. imp. pl.* mix D1032

mery *adj.* happy D264, C264

mesurabely, mesurably *adv.*
moderately D283, D696, C282

mesure *n. owte of* ~ excessively
D989, C989

met(e *n.* food D119, D176, C116.
metis, metys *pl.* D521, C521

methill *see* **medyll**

meve *v.* move D151, C149. **meue,
meve** *imp. pl.* D553, C553.
mevyd(de *pp.* D1006, C1006

myd *adj.* middle, central C70

myddes, myddys *n.* middle, midst
D62, D71, C59

myddyll *adj.* middle D670

myddill, mydyll *n.* waist D638, C638

myddewyffe, mydwyf(fe *n.* midwife,
birth attendant D376, D388, C372

myddilbark *see* **medill bark**

myght, my3ght, my3th, myth *v. pr.
3 sg.* might D191, D252, D397,
C397

mylte *n.* spleen, lungs D147, C146

***mynyster** *v. imp. pl.* administer
D843

mynt(e *n.* mint D732, C732. **myntis**
pl. D748, C748

mirre, myrre *n.* myrrh (*Commiphora
myrrha*) D366, C366, C716

mys *adv.* amiss, wrongly C287

mysgydynge *vbl. n.* misruling,
misconducting C308

mysschapyn, mysshapyn *ppl. adj.*
deformed D273, C273

***myster** *n.* necessity D507

mys-turnyde *ppl. adj.* crippled,
crooked D405

mysturnyng(e, mys-turnynge *vbl. n.*
dislocating, distorting D992,
D1000, C992, C1001

mochil, mochyll *adv.* much D207,
D933

mo(o *adj.* more D11, *D359, C10

moder(e, modyre, mooder, moodir
n. mother D391, D428, C391,
C470, C500; uterus D924.

modere, modyre, modyrs, modris, moodris *n. poss.* D297, D302, D471, C297, C302

moistour, moyster, moystour(e, moysture *n.* moisture D73, C72, C161, C818, C1001

monyth(e *n.* month D101, D104, C101

moodir-wort *n.* motherwort, mugwort, meadowsweet C830

morell *n.* black nightshade D958, C1037

morn, morvn(e, morvnne *n.* morn, morning D642, D737, D787, C788

moroue, morwe *n.* morning D1072, C642

morre *adv.* more D926

mortall *adj.* mortal, deadly D102

mostelion, mustelyon *n.* musk oil D558, C558

moton *n.* mutton D1099

mov, mow *v. pl.* may D8, D340, C993

movth(e, mouthe, mowth(e *n.* mouth, opening D57, D261, D318, C55, C317, C386

mugwort(e, mvgwort *n.* mugwort, motherwort, wormwood *Artemisia)* D738, D786, C735, C786

multiplie, multiply *v.* multiply D3, C3

muske *n.* musk D557

muste *n.* must, wine-dregs C557

mustelyon *see* **mostelion**

namely, namly *adv.* especially, specifically D12, C10

nardileo, nardilion *n.* oil of spikenard D558, C558

narov, narwe *adj.* narrow, constricted D211, C210

nase therlys *n. pl.* nostrils C582

nature *n.* strength, physical constitution D719, C720

navill, navyl(l *n.* navel D50, C49, C56, C59, umbilical chord D453, C453

necessite, necessyte *n. of ~* necessarily D192, C191

necke, nek, nekk(e *n.* neck D57, D346, C54, C347; cervix D317, C316

nedfull *adj.* necessary D275, C742

nedir *adj.* nether, lower C194

nedys *adv.* necessarily D134

nepte *n.* cat-mint, catnip D563, C563

ner *adv.* nearly C587

nethyll, nettill *n.* nettle D655, C573. **netlys** *pl.* D573

nev, new *adj.* new D657, D1067, C655

neygh, ny *adv.* near D292, D879, C291

nygh *adj.* close D261, C261

nitrun *n.* natron, lye, potash D871

noyand, *noyant *adj.* harmful D198, C238

noyeth *v. pr. 3 sg.* harms, hurts C197

noyse, noysse *n.* noise D999, C999

noosse, nose, nosse *n.* nose D217, D553, D577, C216

norce, norys(se, norse *n.* wet nurse D477, D486, C477, C490. **norcis** *pl.* C486

norce, norche, norysh, norsch(e *v.* nurse, rear, nourish D64, D466, D502, C466, C502. **norschyth, noryshith** *pr. 3 sg.* D186, C184. **norished, norschyde** *pp.* D115, C61. **norishynge, norschynge** *ppl. adj.* D495, C494

not(e *n.* nut D366, C366

nother *adv.* neither C150

nowth *adv.* not D949

nutre *n.* ?nitre C729

oblayes, oblees *n. pl.* small cakes or wafers D689, C688

ofte *adj.* frequent D508, C507

oftyre *adv. comp.* more often D507

oftener *adv. comp.* more often C507

ofte tyme, oftvn tyme *adv. phr.* often D225, C224

oyle, oly *n.* D957, C956. ~ *bene-dictum* blessed oil C1071; ~ **ceprine, *cypryne,* ~ *ciperyn, cyperyn* oil of galingale (*Ciperus longus*) or henna shrub D284, D945, C283, C945, C1008; ~ *de bay, de *bavme, de bawme, of … laury, laurion, lavryon* bay oil D388, D550, D591, C387, C551, C591; ~ **mirton, *mirtyn* myrtle oil D284–5, C283; ~ *of lyly* lily oil C1072; ~ *olyf(f, oleve, of olyue* olive oil D284, D387, C283, C387; ~ *roset* rose oil D746, C743

oynementis, oynementys, onymentis *n. pl.* ointments D289, D387, C288

oynyns, oynons, onyons *n. pl.* onions D1031, D1057, C1031

ok(e *n.* oak D328, C616

oliues, olyuys *pl.* olives D557, C557

on, oon *pn.* one D110, D532, C108

on, oo *adj.* one D351, D435, C348, C435

oncurabill, vncurabill *adj.* incurable C109, C243

ony *see* **eny**

onys *adv.* once D101, C101

*opyon *n.* opium, dried juice of green poppy heads D1008

oppressith, oppressyth, op-pressyth *v. pr. 3 sg.* presses on D165, D587, C149

or *conj.* before D253

ordende *v. pa. t.* decreed D3.

ordend(e, ordeyned *pp.* ordained C32, C193; arranged D63, C60

otherwhile, othir-while, othirwhile, oþer-whyll, oþer-whyle *adv.* sometimes D153, D205, C151, C205, C862

othyr(e, outher, outhir *conj.* either D111, D254, C108, C255

otys *n. pl.* oats D570

ouer-hard, ouyre-hard *adj.* excessively hard D263, C263

ouer-hy(e *adv.* excessively high D140, C141

ouer-lov, ouer-lowe *adv.* excessively low D155, C155

ouer-mech(e, ouer-moche *adj.* excessive D227, C226, C227

ouer-mekill *n.* excess C245

ouer-mykyl, ouer-mokyll *adj.* excessive D163, C161

ouer-repleet, ouer-replet(e *adj.* overfull D265, C319, C889

ouer-strait, ouer-streyte *adj.* excessively tight D280, C279

ouerthwart, ouer-thwert, ouyrthwart *adv.* transversely D346, D430, C347

ouyre-owtragisly *adv.* excessively D240

ovyre *see* **howr**

owhte *v. pr. 3 sg.* ought C274

pacient, pacyent *n.* patient, sufferer D170, D784, C168. **pacyentys** *pl.* D948

payne, paynn(e, peyne *n.* pain D540, D584, D911, D960, C911

paynyth, peyneth *v. pr. 3 sg.* pains, hurts D907, C907. **peynynge** *vbl. n.* C822

palasye, palsy *n.* palsy D984, C984

papauere, papauery *n.* poppy
D1004, C1004

pappis, pappys *n. pl.* breasts, nipples
D46, D287, C45, C605

parch *v.* roast, dry D570

parell, perel(l *n.* peril, danger D575,
D886, C575, C884. *oon my ~* at
the risk of damnation D137

parlous, perlous *adj.* dangerous
D947, C948

parsly, persely *n.* parsley D782,
D789

parte, party *n.* part D61, C58; *a ~* in
part C493. **parties, partyes,
partis, partys** *n. pl.* parts D230,
D993, C230, C275, C879

partid, partyde *v. pp.* divided D60,
C57

passe *v.* pass away, die D110; flow
D126, C126. **passith, passyth** *pr.
3 sg.* D157, C157, C854. **passe,
passun, passvn** *pr. pl.* pass D74,
D233, C123

passyngely *adv.* surpassingly,
exceedingly D119, C116

pece, pese *n.* piece, fragment D462,
C461. **pecys** *pl.* D372

pelettis, pelotis *n. pl.* pellets, pills
D760, C760

penne, pynne *n.* feather D590, C590.
pynnys D830

pepir, pepyre *n.* pepper D748, C749

peraventour, peraventure *adv.*
perhaps D344, C345

percell, percill *n.* parsley C782,
C790

perysshith, *peryschyth *pr. 3 sg.*
perishes, dies D71, C70. **perysch,
perish** *pr. pl.* D357, C356.
peryche *subj.* D66

peritory, perytory *n.* pellitory-of-
the-wall (*Paritoria diffusa*) D685,
C685

perterych *n.* partridge D1098

pessary, pissari, pissary(e, pyssary
n. pessary, suppository D557,
C557, C719, C787, C872.
pessarys, pissaries *pl.* D837,
C837

pyntyll *n.* penis C46

place, plase, plasse *n.* place, position
D140, D1006, C140

plaistir, plaster, plastir, plastre *n.*
plaster, poultice D568, D631,
C631, C1048. **plaistris, plastrys**
pl. D289, C288

play, pley *n.* sexual play D264, C264

playn(ne, pleyn *adj.* smooth D55,
C53; open D1067, C1065

**plantayne, plantaynne, playnteyn,
planteyn, plaunteyn, plauntyn** *n.*
plantain D607, D814, C606, C621,
C623, C627

plener(e *adv.* completely D58, C55

pochydde *ppl. adj.* poached D1100

poynt(e *n. in good ~* in good
condition D497, C496–7; *~ of
here herte* location of her heart
D91–2, C92

poliarcon, poliarton *n.* soothing
ointment D870, C869

**polipodye, polypodye, polypodin,
polipodium** *n.* polipody, oak fern
(*Polipodium vulgare*) D327, D616,
C327, C616

pollucion, polucyon *n.* nocturnal
emission D37, C36

pomegarnet, pome granat *n.*
pomgranate D622, C623

poore *adj.* inadequate C120

popy *n.* poppy C652

***pores, pooris, powrys** *n. pl.* pores
D498, D505, C498

portenaunce, portynavns *n.*
appertenances D47, C47

porret *n.* leeks C748

posteme *n.* abcess C1025

potage *n. ryse* ~ rice stew D1089

pouce, *powls, pulse *n.* pulse D539, D545, C539

poudere, poudir, poudyre, povdyre, powder, powdir, powdyre *n.* powder D574, D622, D763, D1072, C574, C623, C637, C725

poure, povere, povyre, pouere, power *n.* power D198. *of* ~ having the ability D123, D237, D510, C510; *at his* ~ as far as possible C197

*preparatyue *n.* preliminary medication D376

precipitacion, precipitation, precipytacion, precypytacion, precipitacyon *n.* prolapse D88, D95, D531, D806, C88

preef, prefe *n.* proof D693, C692

prefocacion, prefocacyon *n.* dislocation D88, D95, C88

preue, preve, proue *v.* test D639, C639, C692. **provyd** *pp.* C366

preuydde, preuyde, provyd, prouyd *ppl. adj.* tested D365, D777, D1040, D1074, C1039

preuy, prevy *adj.* ~ *membris, membrys* genitals D891, C891

prikkyng, prykynge *vbl. n.* pricking, pain D933, C933. **prikkyngis, prykkyngis, prykyngis** *pl.* sharp pains D861, D1011, C860

priuite, priuyte, pryuite, pryuyte, privite, pryvite *n.* D1084, C49, C60, C73, C881; ~ *of the wombe* vagina C48, C262. **preuytees, prevites** *n. pl.* secrets D28, C28

profyrre *v.* offer D693

profitabill, profitabull *adj.* profitable, useful D178, D776, C177

propir, propyr *adj.* appropriate D777, C777

propirly *adv.* appropriately C105

prowde *adj.* proud D314, C313

ptisan, ptysanne *n.* tisane D625, D966

pulial(l, puliol(l *n.* D724, C723, C782; ~ *ryall, riall* pennyroyal, wild thyme D675, C673, C732

purgacion, purgacioun, purgacyon *n.* purgation, purification D200, D682, C200; menstruation D485, C673; post-partum flow D472

purge *v.* purge, purify D199, C198; *refl.* begin to menstruate D690, C689. **purgid, purgyd(e, purgyt** *pp.* D102, D260, C101, C260

purs(e *n.* bag, purse D637, C637

put *v.* push D444, C443. **put** *imp. pl.* ~ *to* place on D378. **puttynge** *vbl. n.* thrusting D292

quakyn, qwakyn *v. pr. pl.* shake, tremble D589, C589, C599

queen, quene, qween *n.* queen D740, C737, C739

quyck, quyk, qwyk, *adj.* alive D362, C365; live, glowing D578, C578

radyk, radysch *n.* radish D764, C764

raynes, raynyes, *raynys, reynes, reynys *n. pl.* kidneys, loins D96, D332, D943, C96, C876

receyt *n.* medicinal recipe, prescription D692

receyue, receyve, reseyf, reseyue, resseyue *v.* receive D6, D63, C5, C60, C576. **receyuyth, resseyuyth** *pr. 3 sg.* D133, C188. **receyue, receyve, resseyue** *pr. 3 pl.* D125, D177, C121. **receyuyd** *pp.* C132. **receyve, resseyue** *subj.*

D977, C977. **recevynge** *vbl. n.* D136

recouer, recovyre *v. trans.* restore, regain D488, C488

rasere, rasour *n.* razor D459, C459

red(e *adj.* red D234, C233

rede *n.* blood-colour C1073

rede, reede *v.* read D20, C19, C20. **rede, reede** *subj,* D25, C25

redy *adj.* prompt D324, C324; unmistakable, clear D1000, C1000

redresse *v.* correct D995, C995

reggebon *n.* spine C159. **ryge-bonys** *poss.* D159

rehersid *ppl. adj.* repeated C219

reynes, reynys *see* **ranys**

reyse, rise, ryse, rysse *v.* arise D129, D586, D940, C125, C586. **reyseth, risith, rysit(h, rysyth(e** *pr. 3 sg.* D140, D288, D859, C102, C140, C539. **rysen, rysyth, ryson** *pr. pl.* D538, D880, C538

releve *v. subj.* get up, recover D95

religios *n. pl.* religious, women under vows D120

religious *adj.* ~ *women* women under vows, nuns C117

remanent, remenavnt, remmenavnt, remnavnt *n.* remaining part D184, D344, D347, C348. **remanentis** *n. pl.* C345

remeved, remewydde *v. pp.* shifted, moved D583, C583

renne, rynne *v.* run D604, C604. **rennyth, rynnyth** *pr. 3 sg.* D493, C1001. **rennyth** *pr. pl.* C860. **renne** *subj.* C492. **rennyng(e, rynnyng** *vbl. n.* D981, C959, C981

rennynge, rynnynge *ppl. adj.* running, flowing D751, C751

repast(e *n.* meal D121, D192, C119

replet(e *adj.* full C265, D889

resistence, resistens *n.* resistance D74, C74

resnabill, resonabill, resonabyll, resonabull *adj.* rational, capable of reason D2, D8, C2; natural D220, C218

reson(ne, reasoun *n.* reason D53, D141, *of ~* according to nature D322, C322

resonabyly, resonably *adv.* naturally, normally D249, D341, C341

restely, restly *adv.* restfully D268, C268

retencion, retencioun, retencyon *n.* D89, D172, C89, C174 retention

reupontyk, rupontijk *n.* rhubarb root (*Rheum rhaponticum*) D789, C789

rew(e, rue, rve, rwe *n.* rue D576, D732, D786, D871, C576

ry3ht, right *adj.* right-hand D81, C81; proper, suitable D313

right, rygth, ry3ght, ry3th, ryht, ryth *adv.* just, exactly D7, D296, D297, D498, C6; ~ *foorth, forth* directly, straight out D380, C380

rynde *n.* bark D670

ripe, *rype, ryppe *v.* cause to come to a head D1050, C1050, C1058. **rypyd** *pp.* D1034

ryse *n.* rice D1089

roses, rosis, rosys *n. pl.* roses D921, C919. ~ *eglente, eglentyn* briar roses D620, C620

rosyn *n.* pine sap, resin D836, C835

rot(e *n.* root D566, D1081, C610. **rootis, rotis, rotys** *n. pl.* D327, C326, C627, C1044

rot(e *v.* cause to rot D528, C528. **rotyth** *pr. 3 sg.* D490. **rote, rotyth** *pr. pl.* D75, C74. **rotyn, rottvn**

intr. rot D196, C195. **rotydde,** *pp.*
D1062

rotyn *adj.* rotten, putrid C1061

rowgh, rowh *adj.* rough D55, C52

rupontijk *see* **reupontyk**

sad(e *adj.* hard D118, C115

saf, saue *prep.* except D681, C679

saffre, saffron, safrvnne, saffvrne *n.*
saffron D708, D835, D842, C707,
C834

sayntys, seyntis, seyntys *n. pl.* saints
D13, D30, C13

salt(e *adj.* salted D528, C527

saltfysch, saltfysh *n.* salt-water fish
D798, C798

salues, salvys *n. pl.* ointments
D1035, C1035

sandragon, sandregragon *n.*
'dragon's blood', red gum,
resin D623, C624

saraseta *see* **trifera**

sauge, savge, sawge *n.* sage (*Salvia
officinalis*) D733, D781, C733,
C781, C790

savayn(e, saveyn(e *n.* savin,
soapwort (*Juniperus sabina*)
D670, D677, C669, C674

saverynge *ppl. adj.* smelling D828

savird, sauyrd *ppl. adj.* wel ~ sweet
smelling C826, *ill* ~ foul smelling
C827

sauor, sauour, savor(e, savour *n.*
smell D255, D554, D678, C256,
C677

scabios, scabious *n.* scabious D1040,
C1039

scalde, skalde *v. imp. pl.* scald, boil
D334, C333

scalis, scalys *n. pl.* scales D751,
C751; shells D632

scew, schew, schev, shewe *v.*
demonstrate D141, D273, D340,

C340. **shev** *pr. 1 sg.* show D109.
schevyth, shewith *pr. 3 sg.*
displays D354, C341. **schew** *pr.
pl.* D341. **schevyd, shewid** *pp.*
revealed D28, C28. **schew, shewe**
subj. D404, C404, *refl.* appear
D435, C435. **schevynge,
shewyng(e** *vbl. n.* D21, C22, C94

schamfull *adj.* shy, embarassed D314

schapyn *v. pp.* shaped D54

schapp *n.* shape, form D58

schare, scharre, shar(e *n.* groin,
pubic region D944, D997, C943,
C998

scharge *see* **charge**

schavynge *see* **chafyng**

**schepe, scheppe, sheep, shep,
schepis, schepys, shepis** *see*
chepe

schyld(e *see* **chyld**

scholdyre, shuldir, shuldre *n.*
shoulder D401, C400, C401.
scholdrys, shuldris *n. pl.* D392,
C392

***sclarye** *see* **clarye**

sclavndyr, sclavndure, slaundir *n.*
slander D26, D28, C26

sclendyre, slendir *adj.* immature, not
fully grown D980, C980

sclydynge, slydynge *ppl. adj.* mobile,
unstable D56, C53

scrape, scrapp *v. imp. pl.* scrape
D656, C654

scrov, scrow(e, skrowe *n.* scroll,
strip of parchment D369, D372,
D373, C369

se *v.* see D52. **se(en** *pr. pl.* D7, D296,
C7. **se** *subj.* D579. **se(ynne** *pp.*
D77, C76

sece, seesse *v.* cease, stop D638,
C639. **sees** *subj.* D771. **cesith,
cesyth, cessith, sesyth** *v. imp. pl.*

cease, stop D680, D683, C679, C681

secunday *adv.* on the second day C671

secundine, secundyne, secundynne, secvndyn(e, secvndynne *n.* afterbirth D293, D295, D301, D793, D794, D799, C295

sede, seed *n.* sperm, semen D5, C4; (plant) seed D330, C329. **sedis, sedys** *pl.* (female) seeds D559, C559

seyn *v.* say C531. **sayth, seith** *pr. 3 sg.* D768, C769. **seid(e** *pa. t.* C587, C935. **sayd(e, seid, seyd** *pp.* D431, D780, D915, C601, C779

seke, syk(e *adj.* sick D117, D428, C427

seknes, sykenes, syknes(se *n.* sickness D11, D117, C10, C91. **syknesses, syknessis** *pl.* C86, C130

seldyn *adv.* seldom, infrequently D43

selidonye *see* **celidony**

semblabyll *adj.* similar D491

senigrene, senygrene, syngrene, ssenygrene *n.* sengreen, houseleek D609, C608, C712, C811

senevey(n, senevy, senvay *n.* mustard D748, D799, C748, C798

senues *see* **synov**

serracyneise *see* ***trifera***

sese *v. imp. pl.* grasp D389, C389

sesyth *see* **sece**

seth(e *v.* process D188, D1048, C188. **seth(e, sethen** *imp. pl.* boil D610, D1052, C610. **sod, soden, sodyn, sodon, sodune, sothen, sothyn** *pp.* D177, D182, D628, C176, C467, C620, C627; soaked D389, C388

seth(en, syth *conj.* since D187, D530, D663

sevet, sewet, suet *n.* suet, fat D289, D716, C288

sew, sue *v.* follow D334, C332. **sewyn, sue** *pr. pl.* D220, C854. **sew, sue** *subj.* continue D869, C868

shalis, shellis *n. pl.* shells C632, C1005

shame-faste *adj.* shy, embarassed C313

shep *see* **chepe**

syde *n.* page D868

syde *n.* loins, womb C1073. **sydes, sydys** *pl.* sides, edges D59, C56; flanks, hips D60, C56

signe, sygne *n.* symptom C16, D984. **signes, sygnes, synes, synnes** *pl.* signs D15, D303, D501, C303, C806

syn *conj.* since C187

synneve, synov, synow *n.* sinew D142, D1068. **senues, senewes, senewis, synevs, synovys, synovs, synvys, synwys** *pl.* D56, D150, D162, D821, D909, C54, C161, C820

sirep, sirip, sirup(pe, syruppe *n.* syrup (herbs boiled with sugar) D561, D614, D1106, C561, C614

sitte, syt(te *v.* sit D703, D742, C703, C739. **setyn, soton** *pp.* sat on, incubated D653, C653

skalde *see* **scalde**

skyn(ne *n.* membrane D297, D307, C296; skin D940, C940

skrowe *see* **scrov**

slack, slak *adv.* slackly, loosely D279, D286, C285

slakyn, slakkyn *v. pr. pl.* slacken D163, C162, C820

slaknesse *n.* looseness D974, C974

slaundir *see* sclavndyr

slawndrynge *vbl. n.* slandering C28

slen *v. pr. pl.* kill D310. sle *subj.* slaughter D640, C640

smalnes(se *n.* emaciation D946, C947

smyte, smythe *v. subj.* strike, hit D859, C859. smytynge *vbl. n.* D308, C308

softe *n.* pulp C557

softe *adj.* mild D387, C386

softe *adv.* gently D399

sok, sowke *v.* suck D469, C469. sok, sowke *subj.* D512, C511. sokynge, sowkynge *vbl. n.* D525, C525

solys *n. pl.* soles D328, C327

sond *v.* make a noise, echo D860. soundith *pr. 3 sg.* C859

soner(e, sonnere, sunner *adv. comp.* sooner D94, D245, D896, C244, C585, C896

soppe, sowpe *v.* sip, drink D957, C956

sore *adv.* sorely, bitterly C240, hard C941

sorys *n. pl.* sores D1063, C1062

sovnde *v.* swoon D92

sovthyrnwode, sowth-thernwoode *n.* southernwood (*Artemisia abrotanum*) D783, C782

sowe *n.* sow D921, C920

sowke *see* sok

spatill, spetyll *n.* spittle D543, C544

spica celtica, *spicam selticam *n.* celtic spikenard (*Valerian celtica*) D782, C781

spicis, spycys *n. pl.* spices D556, C556

stampe *v.* stamp, pound D686. stampid *pa. t.* D741, C738. stamp(e, stompe *imp. pl.* D328, D631, D699, C327

stampydde *ppl. adj.* pounded D916

stanche, staunche *v. intrans.* cease to flow D652, C652. stanchynge, staunching *vbl. n.* D692, C691

staphisagyre, *stavesakre *n.* stavesacre (*Delphinium staphisagria*) D757, C757

stat(e *n.* condition D478, C478

sterith, steryth *v. pr. 3 sg.* stirs, moves D285, C284. stere *imp. pl.* D1048, C1048. steryd, sterid *pp.* stirred, agitated D270, C270. sterynge *vbl. n.* D272, C272

stermutacion, stermuntacyon *n.* sternutation D580, C580

stev *see* stue

stew, stue *n.* subfumigation, herbal decoction, vapour D677, C675. stvys *n. pl.* stews D1102

sticados *n.* houseleek (*Sempervivum tectorum*) D789, *C789

stille, styll(e *adv.* still, unmovingly D544, D845, C542

stomack, stomak(e *n.* stomach D122, D148, C147. stomakys *pl.* C120

ston(ne *n.* stone D462, C462; *the ~* kidney or gall stone D319, C318

stonde *v.* stand, be C300

stope, stoppe *v. subj.* cease D219, C217. stopyd(e, stopyt, stoppid, stoppyd *pp.* obstructed D209, D451, D601, D774, C209; staunched D245, C244

storak, storax *n.* resin from the styrax tree D708, D803, C802. *see also* estorax

storid *pp.* stored D1, C1

straynabill, streynabill *adj.* violent, forceful D621, C622

strayne, streyne *v.* strain, purify D618, C618

strayte, streyte *adj.* narrow D57, C54

strayte, streyte *adv.* tightly D278, C277

strangelid, strangelyde *ppl. adj.* choked D588, C587

stroyde *ppl. adj.* destroyed D293

struccion *n.* ?soapwort (*Saponaria officinalis*) C581

stue, stw *v.* fumigate D798, C797. **stev** *refl. imp. pl.* inhale vapour D1072

subfumigacion, subfumigacyon, suffumigacion, suffumygacion *n.* subfumigation D678, D922, C556, C676

substans *n.* substance, matter D181

sue *see* **sew**

suell, svell, swelle *v.* swell up, bloat D91, D467, C92. **svellyn, swellen, swellyn** *pr. pl.* D538, C538, C895. **suellynge, swellyng** *pr. p.* D537, C537. **suollyn, swollyn** *pp.* D858, C858

suellynge, swellyng(e *n.* swelling D853, D857, C853, C858

suerly *adv.* surely D110

suet *see* **sewet, svete**

sufficith, suffisith, suffysyth *v. pr. 3 sg.* is sufficient D717, D1107, C717

suffocacion, suffocacyon *n.* (uterine) suffocation, D88, D90, *C87, C91

suffir, suffyre, suffre, suffure *v.* bear, endure D335, D680, C334, C703. ~ *naturally* permit sexual relations C900

sumdel(l *adv.* somewhat D491, C491

sunner *adv. see* **soner(e**

superfluite, superfluyte *n.* excess D73, D175, C72, C244 **superfluytes, superfluiteys, superfluites** *pl.* D193, D196, C192

superhabundance, superhabundaunce *n.* overabundance, superfluity D38, C36, C125

superhabundant *adj.* overabundant D129

superhabundantly *adv.* superabundantly D224, *C239

surfet *n.* excess D974, C974

surfetysly, surfetously, surfetusly *adv.* excessively D105, D643, C104

svete *v.* sweat, perspire D738. **suet** *imp. pl.* sweat D1096

svete, sweet *adj.* sweet, pleasant D522, C522

swelle *see* **suell**

swet *n.* sweat, perspiration D504

swone, swowne *n.* swoon, fainting fit D914, C913

swone, swoune *v.* swoon, faint D546, C93. **swonyn, swowne** *pr. pl.* D900, C899. **swonynge, swovnynge, *swownynge** *vbl. n.* D890, C891, C909

tabour, tabure *n.* drum D860, C860

talent *n.* desire D170, C168; urge D881, C880

talow, talwh *n.* tallow D834, C834

tansay, tansy *n.* tansy, common chrysanthemum D738, C735

taught, tavt *v. pa. t.* taught D726, C726

telle, till *conj.* until D251, C252

temper, tempir, tempyr(e *v. imp. pl.* mix D579, D712, D1008, C579, C723

tempure *n.* blending or mixing in due proportion D6, *C5

tenchys *n. pl.* tenches D1104

tent *n.* surgical drain D1035, C1035

teodoricon, teodoricioun,
theodoricon *n. ~ anacardinum*
D776, C775. *~ empiston,
euperiston* D777, C776 purgative
medicaments

terebentyne, terebentynne,
*terpentine, terpentyne *n.*
terebinth, turpentine (*Pistacia
terebinthus*) D717, D834, C717,
C833

terme *n.* period D680; time of
menstruation C671; *~ of his lyf* for
the duration of his life C513–4

tesan, tisan *n.* tisane, herbal infusion,
barley water D797, C797. tysanys
pl. C625

tesyk, tysyk *n.* pthisis, consumption
D111, C108

tete *n.* nipple, breast D523. tetys
poss. D524

thedir, thedyre *adv.* thither D605,
C604

thenne, thyn *adj.* thin D55, C52

thens, þens *adv.* thence D185, D454,
C183

theys, þeys, thes, þes *pn.* these D108,
D303, D895, C107

theodoricon *see* teodoricon

therouer, þer-ouyre *adv.* above,
over (it) D703, C703

thyck, thykke *adv.* thickly D590,
C590

thyk, thikke *adj.* thickened D985,
C985

thyke heryde, þik herid, *adj.* having
abundant hair D43–4, C43

thyknesse *n.* thickness, viscosity
C212

thyn *see* thenne

thirday *adv.* on the third day C672

thirste, thyrst, threste, thryst *v.*
subj. thrust, press D858, D939,
C858, C939

tho *pn.* those D117, C261

tho(o *adj.* those D30, D193, C30

þorow, throw(h *prep.* through D700,
C700, C819

thosydde, tosid, tosydde *ppl. adj.*
teased D607, D730, C607

thow(gh *conj.* though D936, C328,
C966

threde, threed *n.* thread D454, C454

throwys *n. pl.* contractions, labour
pains D327, C326

thurde *adj.* third D3

tille *n.* tile D1071

tymely *adv.* quickly, promptly C395

tymfull *adj.* timely, seasonable, due
D324

tode *n.* toad D636, C636

token, tokyn *n.* distinguishing mark.
D76, C75

ton *adj.* the one C157

tonge, tunge *n.* language D18, C19,
tongue D589, C589

to(o *adj.* two D634, C210

tooys *n. pl.* toes D1101

tosid, tosydde *see* thosydde

tother, tothir *adj.* the other C82,
C318

tovncrasse *n.* garden cress (*Lepidum
sativum*) D814. ton-cressis,
toncresses, tovncrassys *pl.* D804,
C803, C813

towche, tuche *v.* touch, carress D934,
C934. tochyth *pr. 3 sg.* D150.
toche, towche *subj.* D936, C936

translatid, translatyde *v. ppl*
translated D17, C17

trauayle, travell, travill, travyll *n.*
labour, toil D10, D134, D136, C9

trauayle, trauell, travayle, travell *v.*
labour D483, C360; *trans.* make
work D269. *~ of chylde, child*
labour in childbirth D305, C305.
trauailith, trauaylith, trauelyth,

travelyth *pr. 3 sg.* D326, D441, C326, C339. **trauailed, trauayled, trauelyd** *pp.* D478, C478, C866. **trauelynge, traueylyng, travelynge** *vbl. n.* D87, D647, C87

trees, treys *n. pl.* trees D8, C7

tretys *n.* treatise D17, C17

tretyth *v. pr. 3 sg.* discusses D301

trifera *n.* ~ *saraseta, serracyneise* trifera sarracenica or Saracen trifera, a cleansing medicine D614, C613–4; ~ *magna, the grete* D775, C775

troublith, trovbelyth *v. pr. 3 sg.* troubles, disturbs D169, C167

tweys, twyes *adv.* twice D478, D507, C478

twyk *v. subj.* tweak, pull sharply or suddenly C500

vnc(e, unce *n.* ounce D709, D712, C708, C791

vncurabill *see* **oncurabill**

vndefyed, undefyed *ppl. adj.* undigested D193, C192

vndernethe, vndyrnethe *adv.* below, beneath D718, C719

vndertake, vndyrtak *v.* assume responsibility, commit oneself D666, C664

vnlettyrd, vnlettrid *ppl. adj.* illiterate, unlearned D20, C20

vrinall, vrynall *n.* urine bottle D58, C55

vrine, vryn(e, vrynne, urine *n.* urine D208, C207; *gret(e* ~ fecal matter D157, D166, D168, C157, C164. ~ *symple, sympull* urine D165, C163

vrsyn *n.* acanthus C1051

vse *v.* use, practise D249. ~ *hire body naturaly* have sexual intercourse C249. **vsith, vsyth** *pr. 3 sg.* is

accustomed D820, C818. **vsed, vsydde** *pa. t.* D719, C719. **vsydde** *pp.* D749. **vse** *subj.* C483. **vse** *imp. pl.* accustom D521, C521

vayne, veyne *n.* vein, blood vessel D951, C951. ~ *epatik, epatyk* hepatic vein D603, C603. **vaynes, veynes, waynes** *n. pl.* D211, D538, C212

vastyde *see* **wasteth**

vatyre *see* **water**

vax *see* **wax(e**

veynd *see* **wene**

vengavns, vengeaunce *n.* vengeance, retribution D27, C27

venym *n.* venom, poison D197

ventosse, ventouse *n.* cupping glass D605, C605

vertis *see* **wertis**

vesell, vesyll, vessel(l, vessyll, *n.* organ D51, D55, D70, D126, C50, C52. **vesellys, vesels, vessellis** *pl.* chambers, compartments D60, D69, C57

vyces *n. pl.* ills, complaints D904

vinegir, vyneger, vynegyre, wyneegyre *n.* vinegar D626, D649, C626, C648

vitaill, vytall *n.* food D122, C119

vitrum *n.* ?error for *nitrum*, natron, lye, potash C870

*****voyde, woyde** *v.* expell D237, D239. **voidith, voydith, voydyth** *v. pr. 3 sg.* D197, C197, C237. **woyde** *pr. pl.* D977

voys, woyce *n.* voice, cry D500, C499

vom *n.* foam, vomit D588

vomet, vomyt, womet *n.* vomit D217, D810, C588. **vometis** *n. pl.* vomitings C215

wayys, weyes *n. pl.* ways, methods D111, C215

waynes *see* **veyne**

wake *v. pr. 3 pl.* watch, keep vigil D119. **wakyng(e** *vbl. n.* D120, C118

wamelynge *vbl. n.* nausea, wobbling D947, C947

wantyn *v. pr. 3 sg.* lack C119

war(e *adj.* wary, careful D527, C437

war(e *v. subj.* beware C527, C866

wasch, wash *v.* wash D562, C562. **wasch, washe** *pp.* D506, C507. **wasch** *imp. pl.* D1077. **waschynge, washynge** *vbl. n.* D508, C508

*wasteth, wastith, wastyth *v. pr. 3 sg.* wastes away, diminishes D117, D121, C118. **vastyde, wastyd(de** *pp.* D207, D720, C124

water, watir, watyre, vatyre *n.* urine D215, C214; water D244, C243

watir-lyke, watyre-lycke *adj.* watery D235, C233–4

wax(e, wex(e *v.* D2, D304, C2, C304 grow. ***waxethe, waxith, wexith** *pr. 3 sg.* D906, C906, C929. **wax(en, wex-yn, vax** *pr. pl.* become D163, D880, C162, C879

weche *v. pr. pl.* keep vigil, stay awake C117

wey3te *n.* weight C580

weket, wyket, wikket, wykket *n.* female external genitals D290. ~ *of þe wombe* D49, D50, D77

welde, whilde, whyld(e *adj.* wild D1038, D1057, D1098, C1038

wele, wyle *adv.* well D512, D514

welewyn *n.* error for **wyld vyne** 1091

wene *v¹.* wean C520. **veynd** *pp.* D520

wene *v².* *pr. pl.* think, believe D541, C541

werinesse, werynes *n.* tiredness, exhaustion D946, C946

werke *n.* activity C291

wertis, vertis *n. pl.* warts, pimples D45, C44

wete, whete *v.* wet, moisten D388, C387. **weete, wete** *imp. pl.* D468, C468, C551

wete(n *v.* know D969, C968. **wethyth, wit** *v. imp.* D374, C370. **wete** *subj.* D514

wete-mel, whete-mele, whete-melle *n.* wheatmeal D629, D1031, C629

wex(e *n.* wax D972, D1006

whedir, *whethyre *conj.* whether D362, C362

whete *n.* wheat D687

whight, white *n.* white (of an egg) D842, C841, C920

whight, whyght, white, whyte, whytte *adj.* white D671, D700, D1004, C700, C707, C830

whynne, wyne, wyn(ne *n.* wine D367, D1005, D1058, C367, C670

whoman *n.* woman D19. **whomen** *pl.* D9. **womanys, womannys, womans** *poss.* D85, D96, D238

whombe, wombe *n.* stomach D465; belly D283, D833, C282; womb, uterus D49, C48

wichcrafte, wyche-crafte *n.* witchcraft D463, C463

wyf *n.* woman C1070

wyket, wikket, wykket *see* **weket**

wyldemalwe *n.* wild mallow C1044

wyll, wol(l *v. pr. 1 sg* will, intend D85, D531, D532. **wol, wule** *pr. 3 sg.* D136, D940. **wol(l** *pl.* D295, D558. **wolde** *pa. t.* would, requires D53, would like to D78

wympyls, wymplis *n. pl.* head coverings, wimples D956, C955

wyneegyre *see* **vinegir**

wyntyr *n.* winter, i.e. year D108

wys *adj.* careful C437

wysely *adv.* carefully C382

wyt *see* **weten**

with-hold, withholdyn *v. pp.* withheld, retained D989, C208

with-in, with-jnne *adv.* inside D404, C404

with-jnfoorth, with-inforth *adv.* within D619, C619

woyce *see* **voys**

woyde *see* **voyde**

wol(l *see* **wyll**

woll(e, wulle *n.* wool D331, D893, C330

wombe *see* **whombe**

womet *see* **vomet**

wond(e, wound(e *n.* wound D965, D969, C964, C991, C1042. **wondys, woundes, woundys** *pl.* D585, C585, C1036

wonder, wondure *n.* miracle D94, C94

wont(e *ppl. adj.* accustomed D461, D668, C461

workyth *v. imp. pl.* do, act D82

wormood, wormwode *n.* wormwood D562, C562

worschyp, worship *n.* honour D13, C13

wrap, wrapp(e *v. imp. pl.* wrap D778, D786, C778. **wrappede** *pp.* D296

wrapped, wrappid, wrappyde *ppl. adj.* wrapped, enclosed D297, C297

wrathfoll, wrathfull *adj.* wrathful, angry D480, C481

wryht, wryt(e, wryth *v.* write D311, D325, D754, D1014. **wreten, wrytyn, wryttyn** *pp.* D22, D868, C22. **write, wryt** *imp. pl.* D369, C369

wrynge *v. imp pl.* wring, squeeze D567, C686

yeer, yere *n.* year D107, C105

yello *n.* yellow, yolk (of an egg) C1055

yelew, yelov *adj.* yellow D233, C232

yerde *n.* penis D47

yes *see* **eyen**

yeue *v.* give C508. **yeue** *pr. pl.* C486. **yeue** *imp.* D360, C363. **yeue** *subj.* D721 *see also* **geve**

yif(f, ȝif(f, yf *conj.* if D377, D429, D648, C24, C477

ȝolk *n.* yolk, yellow (of an egg) D1054

yong(e *adj.* young D124, D477, C122, C477

your(e, yower, yowur *poss. adj.* your D378, D577, C379, C577

zimia *n.* kind of abcess D1020, C1020